FASHION HELP
FOR EVERY WOMAN

GLAMOUR'S
BIG BOOK OF DOS & DON'TS

CINDI LEIVE
& THE EDITORS OF GLAMOUR

WITH TEXT BY
REBECCA SAMPLE GERSTUNG

DESIGN BY
NUMBER SEVENTEEN, NYC

PUBLISHED BY
GOTHAM BOOKS

PRODUCED BY
MELCHER MEDIA

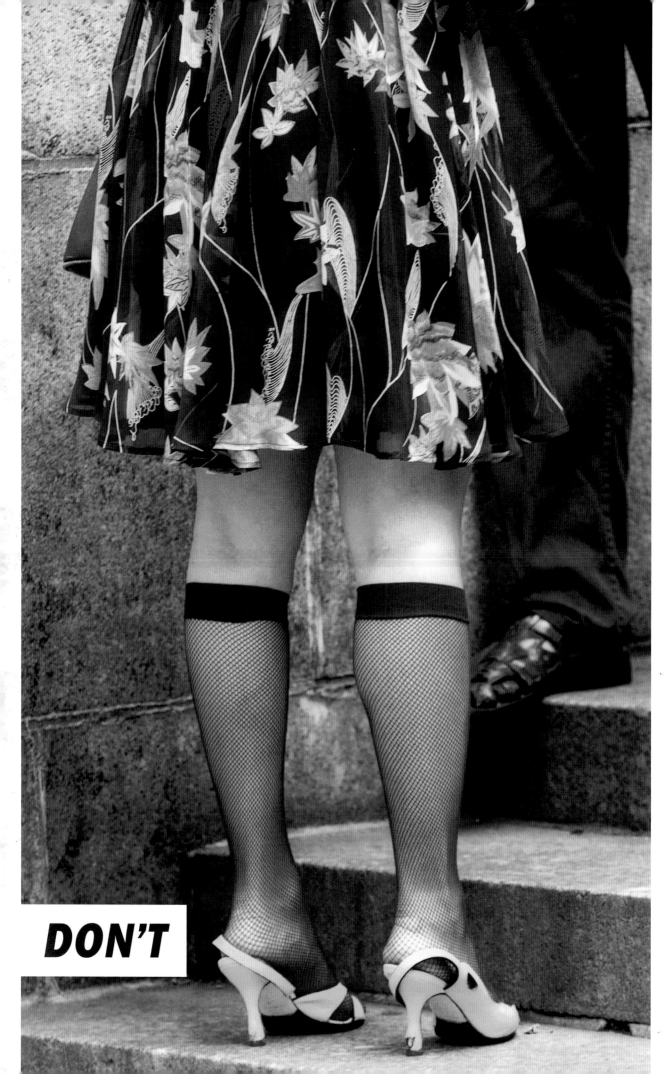

DON'T

contents

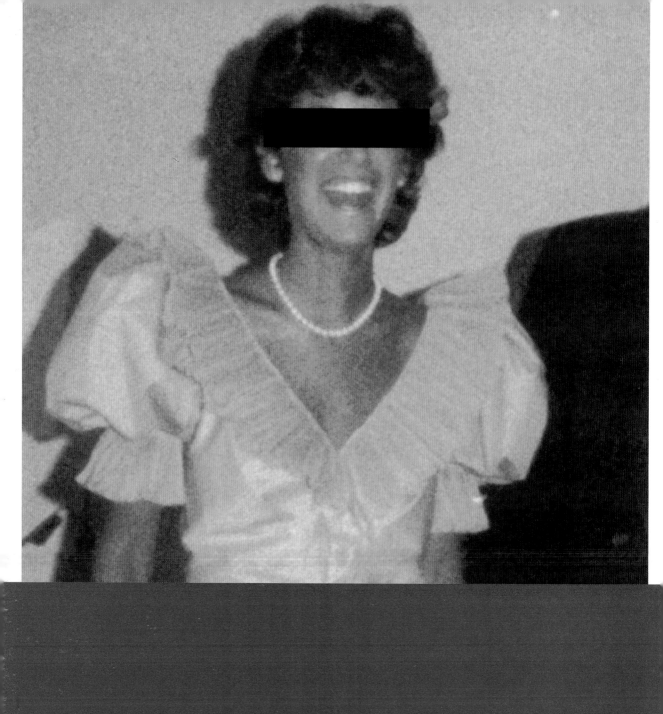

ME IN THE MOST
BEAUTIFUL PROM DRESS
I'D EVER SEEN, CIRCA
1984. THE MUTTON-CHOP
SLEEVES, THE BLINDING
ELECTRIC TEAL, THE
FLAMMABLE TAFFETA—
WHAT WAS I THINKING? IT'S
A TRIPLE-THREAT DON'T!

introduction

CINDI LEIVE, EDITOR IN CHIEF OF *GLAMOUR*

No one **WANTS** to be a *Glamour* Don't.
No one **TRIES** to be a *Glamour* Don't.
In fact, appearing on the back page of
Glamour with a black bar over your eyes
is about the last thing any of us is going
for when we get dressed in the morning.

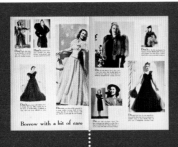

A great idea is born! The first issue of *Glamour* is published, with the first Dos & Don'ts section. Devoted to Hollywood stars, tips range from the always-true "Don't get too fussy with feathers" to the not-as-evergreen "Do take a bright evening tip from Olivia de Havilland and have an embroidered chiffon kerchief to top your hair."

1939

But let's get one thing straight:
WE'VE ALL HAD OUR DON'T DAYS.

Demi Moore showed up in bike shorts at the Oscars one year, and even Gwyneth Paltrow had her pink suede pants split up the back at a movie premiere. Perfectly stylish women have, in their weaker sartorial moments, overdone the animal print theme, found themselves fatally attracted to spandex and strolled out of restrooms with their hems caught in their waistbands.

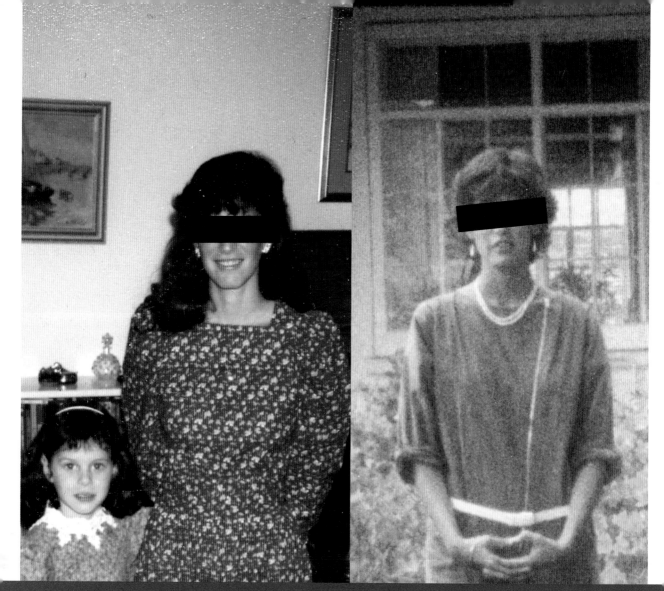

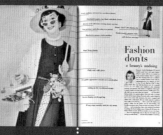

Glamour dresses up TV actress Gisèle MacKenzie as the ultimate Don't. Some of the taboos are timeless—visible slip, dark hose with open-toed mules—but others are not, like the ban on chokers in the summer (According to *Glamour*: "A choker makes a hot day feel even hotter." Not true!)

1957

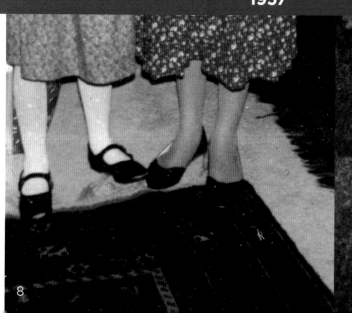

LEFT: LAURA ASHLEY OVERLOAD! I'M 21 HERE. THOSE SWEET LITTLE FLORALS WERE A DO ON MY THEN SIX-YEAR-OLD SISTER, A DON'T ON GROWN-UP ME.

RIGHT: THIS WAS MY FLOCK OF SEAGULLS MOMENT. IT'S A JUMPSUIT WITH AN ASYMMETRICAL ZIPPER THAT WENT UP ONE LEG AND CROSSED TO MY OPPOSITE SHOULDER. SOMETIMES IT'S IMPOSSIBLE TO SEE PAST YOUR OWN DON'TNESS AT THE TIME.

Me? I edit a fashion magazine—and yet, on one sorry morning in 1990, the thigh-high stockings a fashion-editor friend had persuaded me to buy completely collapsed as I rushed through New York City's Grand Central Station. (I kicked them off, balled them up, stuck them in the closest trash can—and crossed my fingers that *Glamour*'s photographers were nowhere nearby.) What can I say? We've all made fashion mistakes. But now, with the help of this book, we'll make many fewer.

Glamour's Dos & Don'ts began in the very first issue of the magazine, back in 1939, though you'd be unwise to act on the advice we offered then. (We proclaimed hairnets a Do. Oops!) But in the almost 70 years since then, we've tried to offer real fashion help for real women. That's the point of Dos & Don'ts, after all—to learn from others' style slipups. It's hard to believe that some of the Don't outfits we've featured actually made it out of the house, but they did—and they still do all the time.

These days our roving photographer, Ronnie Andren, shoots an average of 400 rolls of film a month. That's more than 170,000 photos a year! We've sent him across the country and back several times over, to cities big and small—Seattle; Santa Fe; Denver; Lincoln, Nebraska; Las Vegas; San Francisco and even Lansing, Michigan. He's covered fashion shows, Nascar races, spring break, music festivals and political conventions. Nobody is safe from his lens—not

THREE FASHION MANTRAS TO REPEAT:

1. IT'S NOT ABOUT YOUR BODY.
Whether you're a curvy plus-size or a petite string bean, you don't have to have a "perfect" body to look perfectly chic. Most stylish women don't have model bodies. The secret to their success is that they know what works for their shape, and they use what they've got to their advantage.

2. IT'S NOT ABOUT YOUR BUDGET.
Take one stroll down Rodeo Drive and you see that money can't buy style. How you put your clothes together matters much more than what you pay for them. And no one needs a monster wardrobe. Have one great suit that fits you like a glove? Wear it every week.

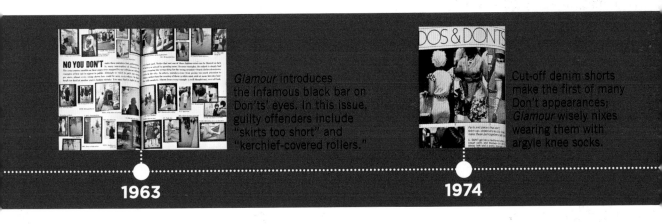

Glamour introduces the infamous black bar on Don'ts' eyes. In this issue, guilty offenders include "skirts too short" and "kerchief-covered rollers."

1963

Cut-off denim shorts make the first of many Don't appearances; *Glamour* wisely nixes wearing them with argyle knee socks.

1974

even me. I was actually snapped on the street before I worked at *Glamour*. Luckily, he got me on a Do day!

Ronnie says that for every Do he sees on the street, he spots five Don'ts—and now we're sharing those real-life pictures with you, plus lots of snaps of models in their off-stage clothes and juicy pix of celebs at their faaabulous best and, well, other times, too.

So gasp, point, laugh out loud (it's impossible not to) and then read on, because there's a Do message within every Don't: Seeing an example of what doesn't work always helps us figure out what does.

3. IT *IS* ABOUT YOUR ATTITUDE
If you walk like a million bucks, you'll look like a million bucks—simple as that. Get rid of any items in your closet that undermine your confidence: If just seeing it on your hanger reminds you that you don't have the hips or the social life for it, then give it to your favorite charity (mine is Dress for Success) and move on.

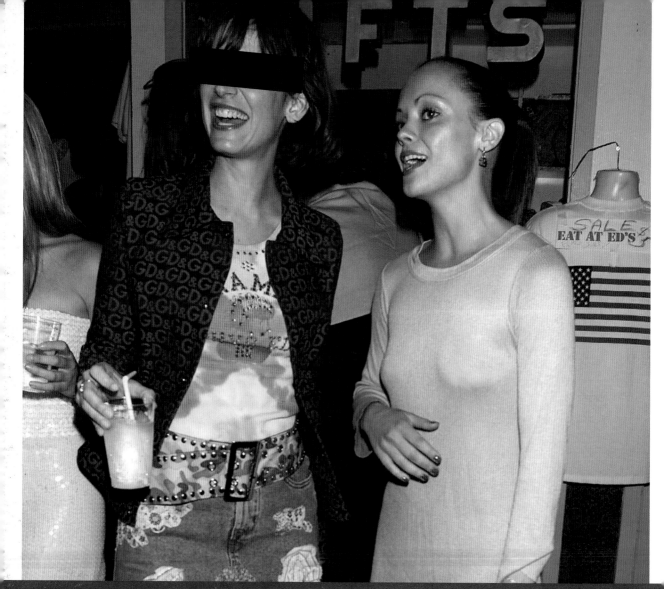

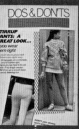

DOS & DON'TS

TIRRUP
ANTS: A
REAT LOOK...
you wear
em right

Eager *Glamour* readers find themselves reading the magazine backward. Dos & Don'ts moves to the final page, its spot today.

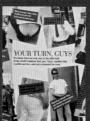

YOUR TURN, GUYS

Finally! *Glamour* calls men on their style crimes: butt cleavage, too many chains and even VBL (visible brief lines).

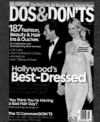

DOS&DON'TS

187 Fashion, Beauty & Hair Ins & Ouches

Hollywood's
Best-Dressed

Glamour comes out with its first special issue dedicated to Dos & Don'ts; eternal Do Claudia Schiffer is on the cover (she's on page 83 of this book).

1985   **1991**   **2000**

AND THE DON'TS KEEP COMING!

ME, *LEFT*, AT A GLAMOUR DON'T PARTY, WHERE EVERYONE IS ENCOURAGED TO COME AS A DON'T. IT'S THE ONE NIGHT OF THE YEAR NOT TO WORRY ABOUT WHAT YOU LOOK LIKE—WORSE IS BETTER. LIKE MY LOGO OVERLOAD?

Of course, getting dressed isn't just about following rules. This book will encourage you to hone your own personal style and stick with it. We're also pleased to announce that the fashion police are relaxing these days; what was a Don't years ago is often a Do today. So next time your mother calls you out for wearing white pants in October or jeans to work, show her "The New Rules" on page 12.

That said, there are some eternal truths to dress by. Some that help me when I'm standing in front of my closet in the morning are:

- The bare-skin thing only works in Hollywood. Those pictures you see everywhere of Paris Hilton or Tara Reid with their bellies showing and their thongs hanging out? No one with a business card should be caught dead in that look. (I recently conducted a job interview where the applicant was wearing a tube top—a tube top!) When in doubt, button up.

- Splurge for the highest quality you can on the true style essentials, which in my mind can be boiled down to this simple list: a great black dress, a killer pair of jeans, a knockout coat, one pair of bright, stylish shoes and a bag that at least looks expensive (and if it wasn't, good for you). Build on these at whatever prices work for you.

- At work, heed the words of a former boss of mine: "Sometimes you have to dress up—just to remind people that you can." Even if it's perfectly acceptable to do your job in jeans and sneaks, it's worth making an effort once in a while. Dress like a honcho, and people are more likely to see you as one.

Fashion isn't rocket science, but it can take some thought and planning to figure out what looks best. That's where *Glamour's Big Book of Dos & Don'ts* comes in. We're here to provide usable advice, wardrobe must-haves, inspiring makeovers, some good laughs and some guaranteed jaw-dropping Don'ts. If you're one of our many anonymous Dos, congrats! (Unknown Do woman on the cover: We photographed you three years ago on a New York City sidewalk, and you still look great to us now.) And if you recognize yourself hiding under a black bar, remember, we're laughing with you, not at you. We've all looked down or looked back (see my prom picture, page 6, for proof) and felt mortified. Like a trusted friend who'll tell you if you ever get spinach stuck between your teeth, *Glamour* is here to help you avoid those moments.

Read on and be Don't-proof!

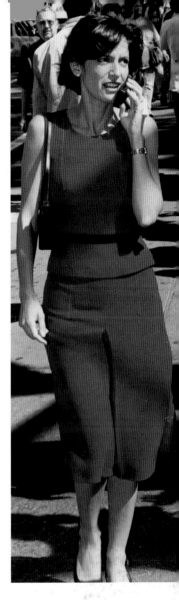

NEED PROOF OUR DOS & DON'TS ARE REAL? OUR ROVING PHOTOGRAPHER ONCE SNAPPED ME ON THE STREET BY ACCIDENT (TOP).

HERE I AM WITH THE UN-DON'T-ABLE SARAH JESSICA PARKER (BOTTOM).

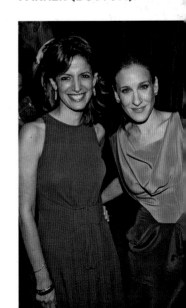

THE {NEW} RULES

Just like clothes, style laws have gotten less uptight and more down-to-earth. Enjoy your new freedom!

NO, YOUR SHOES AND BAG *DON'T* HAVE TO MATCH.

The old matchy-matchy look is over. These days shoes, belts and bags are so wondrously unique that they don't have to go together. Choose them based on what complements your outfit—or delights your eyes.

YES, YOU *CAN* WEAR TWO PATTERNED PIECES TOGETHER.

Paisley and stripes? Florals and gingham? Absolutely! Mix up two prints for an individual, bohemian look. The secret to keeping your outfit chic (and not headache-inducing): Choose pieces in the same color family.

WHITE CLOTHES LOOK GREAT ALL YEAR ROUND.

Forget that old idea that you have to lock them away after Labor Day. As long as the fabrics are appropriate to the climate and season (i.e., no white linen in December), you're good to go. And P.S.: White jeans are a 12-month DO.

WEARING BLACK AT WEDDINGS ISN'T BAD LUCK—IT'S CHIC!

You won't be casting a hex on the newlyweds. This former Don't is now a common, no-brainer Do at evening nuptials, because of the brilliant ubiquity of the Little Black Dress.

PREGNANT? YOUR CLOTHES SHOULD DISPLAY THAT BUMP, NOT COVER IT UP.

Thanks to great maternity designers and countless belly-proud celebs, "stylishly pregnant" isn't an oxymoron anymore. That means even at eight months you can wear pretty much the same stuff you've always loved: cool jeans, fitted tees, sexy skirts, even bikinis.

YOU DON'T *HAVE* TO WEAR A SUIT.

The old suit-at-work law arose at a time when women felt that they had to dress like men to be respected. Today, the best suits have feminine details—if you even want to wear one at all. Sweater sets, skirts and coat and sheath combos are just as appropriate. Heck, even Condoleezza Rice wears dresses!

SOME LINGERIE IS TOO PRETTY TO HIDE.

A peek of lace under a blouse, a cami in place of a shell, or a vintage-y nightgown as a slipdress aren't risqué anymore, they're A Look. A pretty, feminine one.

YOU CAN SKIP THE PANTYHOSE.

A freshly shaved, well-moisturized leg is dressy enough. (Tip: If you like how hose make your skin look even, try self-tanner.) The only two stockings-required occasions: if your office mandates them, or if you're meeting with royalty.

COLORS THAT USED TO CLASH NOW LOOK COOL.

Go ahead and pair black and brown, black and navy, even (carefully) red and pink. What once looked like a result of getting dressed in the dark is now (and forever) stylish.

LET YOUR SHAPE SHOW.

Contorting or confining your curves? That's so over. Dress to accentuate the parts you like, and play down the ones you don't. You'll look and feel great—a Do in any decade!

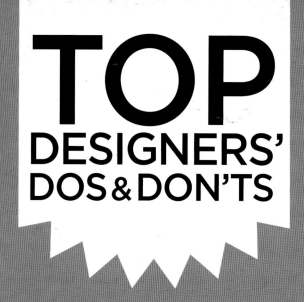

TOP DESIGNERS' DOS & DON'TS

WARDROBE WISDOM FROM THE PEOPLE WHO ACTUALLY MAKE THE CLOTHES. READ AND LEARN!

Isaac Mizrahi:
"Don't wear tons of super-tight clothing. We've been seeing it for so long now, I'm over it! Not to mention that it looks so uncomfortable."

Frida Giannini of Gucci:
"Do pick pieces that reflect your personality instead of following some social sense of what's 'right.' Today it's appropriate to wear jeans with vintage pieces and an evening bag."

Holly Dunlap of Hollywould:
"Don't let your new heels hurt your feet. Take them to the shoe-repair shop and have them stretched a bit so they don't pinch."

Anna Sui:
"Do mix floaty silhouettes like flowy tops, tunics and dresses into your wardrobe; they always feel more free-spirited than an allover tailored style."

Carolina Herrera:
"Do have a signature piece of costume jewelry, like enamel bangles. I can't stop wearing mine."

Malia Mills:
"Do make sure the leg opening of your swimsuit hits the widest part of your hip, not your thigh—makes your legs look longer!"

Jade Jagger:
"Do appreciate the importance of sparkle. My dad taught me that even on days when I want to be comfortable, sometimes it's more fun to be sensational. Jazz it up a bit!"

Nanette Lepore:
"Don't wear a cropped top with low-waisted pants."

Valentino:
"When in doubt, Do wear red. Red is very passionate and sexy. Men go wild for it, and a red with a little bit of orange in it is good on any skin tone."

John Galliano:

"Don't wear what everyone else is wearing. Life's too short to be mundane. Try pairing things that contrast—something very refined with something savage!"

Kari Sigerson of Sigerson Morrison:

"Don't wear your flip-flops with everything. Rely on a pair of smart flats instead, and be stylish and comfortable."

Alexander McQueen:

"Don't wear lacy underwear peeping over the waistband of a pair of jeans; it's not a good look."

Betsey Johnson:

"If you love kooky stuff, Don't wear too many layers. Patterns and prints look best in small doses, and make sure that they fit—too big looks sloppy."

Georgina Chapman of Marchesa: "Do wear a bodyshaper—I love SPANX!—when you want to hide any imperfections."

Roberto Cavalli:

"Don't overdo it. The line between vulgar and sexy is sometimes very thin."

Diane von Furstenberg: "Do learn to be comfortable in your own skin and with what you're doing in your life. If you want to look beautiful, you have to be confident."

AND ADVICE TO DRESS BY FROM GLAMOUR CONTRIBUTOR MICHAEL KORS

DON'T fall for a trend that makes no sense in your life. If you're a city girl, you can get away with wearing glam evening-y pieces for day. But if you've got a super-casual lifestyle, don't bother. You'll just feel silly.

• • •

DO look in a three-way mirror to make sure your pants fit well! I'm amazed by how many women wear unflattering pants.

• • •

DO always wear a great smile—a sense of humor is the sexiest thing in the world.

• • •

DON'T fail to bring some colorful accessories into your life. Really, there are so many gorgeous shoes, bags, belts and sunglasses at every price, you have no excuse not to carry a bright orange bag this once!

• • •

DO try to find your "uniform." To figure out what your go-to outfit is just think about what you always get compliments on.

• • •

DON'T forget that even if you're wearing a dress and heels, you have to be comfortable. If you're in pain and miserable, who's going to flirt with you?

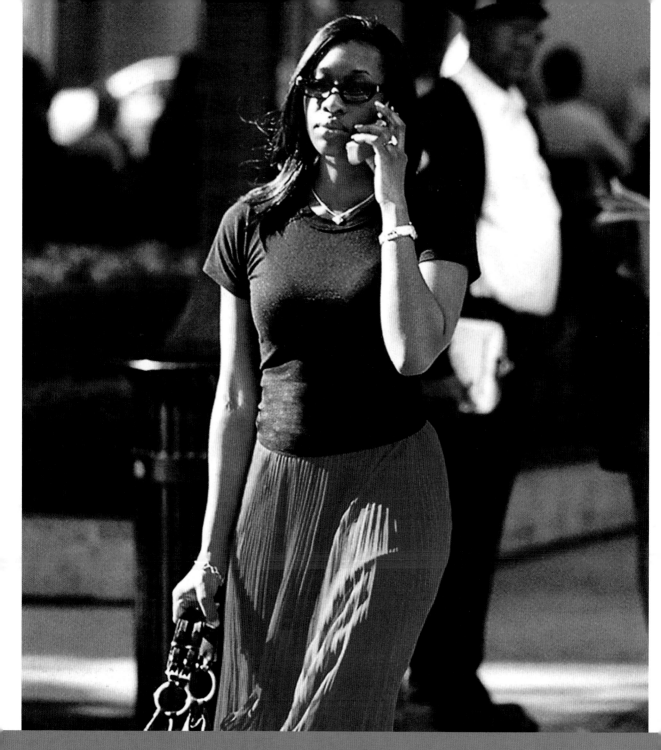

YOUR

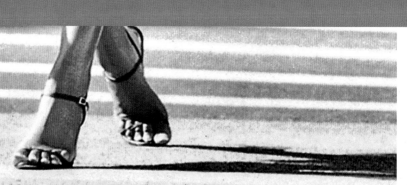

DO

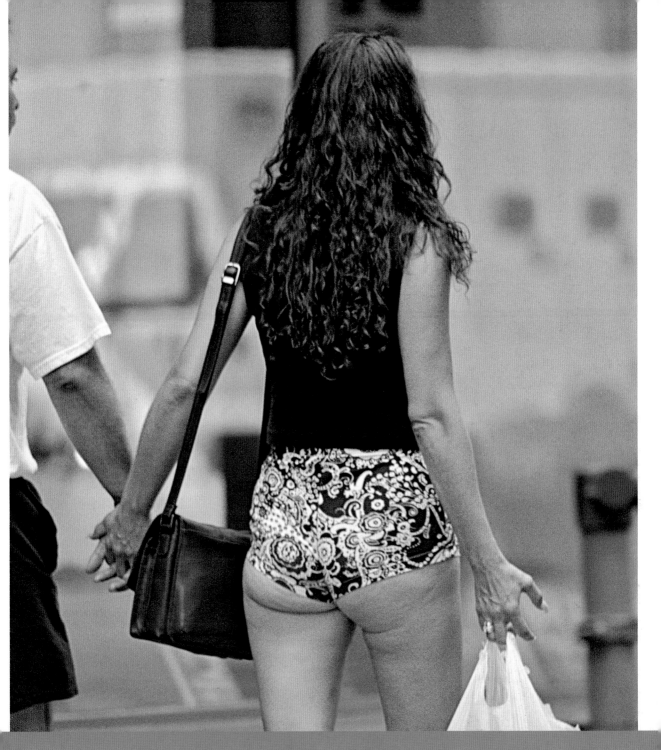

BODY BASICS

ESSENTIAL TIPS & TRICKS TO
DRESS SMARTER FOR *YOUR* SHAPE

DON'T

THE RULES
for flattery

REMEMBER: IT'S ALL ABOUT PROPORTION.

Almost all bodies look better in a mix of fuller and slimmer shapes—a fitted top with a more generous skirt, for instance, or vice versa.

PRACTICE THE ART OF CAMOUFLAGE.

An undisputed fashion truth: Darker colors minimize, and lighter or shiny ones highlight. To play down a double-D chest, avoid wearing bright silver tops. Have a thicker waist? The dark brown belt is better than the white.

SHOWCASE YOUR FAVORITE FEATURE.

Accentuate the positive: Bare tops draw the eye to toned arms; form-fitting jeans highlight your great butt; a V-neck shows off a sexy décolletage divinely.

CHOOSE FIGURE-FLATTERING FABRICS.

When you're trying to de-emphasize a body part, a crisp fabric with some structure is best, like woven cotton or not-stretchy wool. Save clingier fabrics like jersey for areas you want to flaunt.

THE A-LINE IS YOUR FRIEND.

A knee-length A-line skirt or dress (fitted at the hips, looser through the thigh) looks good on almost every body type—especially pear-shapes.

USE PATTERNS WISELY.

Short? Wear a printed top to draw the eye upward. Not curvy? A splashy floral skirt makes a little more of your hips.

KNOW THE POWER OF BEING MONOCHROMATIC.

Wearing the same color, or shades of it, from top to bottom elongates your shape, thinning you out.

IF YOU CAN FOLLOW ONLY ONE RULE, THIS IS IT!

DON'T GO TOO BAGGY—BIG SHAPES MAKE *YOU* LOOK BIGGER.

The muumuu flatters no one! Follow Edith Head's advice, and wear clothes loose enough to prove you're a lady but tight enough to show you are a woman.

TAILOR YOUR CLOTHES TO FIT YOUR INDIVIDUAL SHAPE.

You can't expect every size 12 dress to fit every size 12 woman in the bust, waist and hips. That means you should find a reliable tailor so your clothes fit your body.

REPEAT AFTER US: *ANY* BODY IS A GOOD BODY!

DO or DON'Tness has nothing to do with size. These days, flattering choices abound for women of all shapes. Size 2? Size 22? Dress your body like you respect it.

IF YOU'RE
PEAR-SHAPED...

YOU
have
Smaller shoulders, bust and waist, with heavier hips, bottom and thighs.

YOU
want
To balance your proportions by visually slimming your bottom half and playing up your top.

YOUR
challenge
To become a master of disguise.

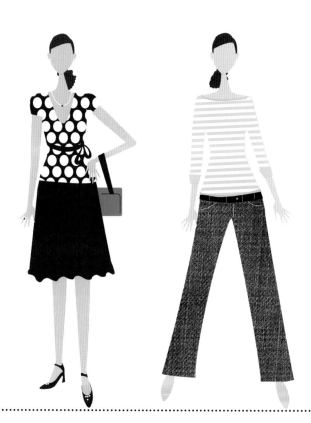

AT WORK
- Detailed, ruffled or colorful tops draw the eye up.
- A dark, A-line skirt with no waistband is ideal.
- Sleek boot-cut or straight pants make hips look narrower.
- Heels are height-inducing and leg-slimming.

ON THE WEEKEND
- A striped boatneck's horizontal line helps balance your top and bottom.
- Look for shirts that hit at the top of the hip-bone.
- On-the-hip boot-cut jeans with biggish pockets are great on your bum.

YOUR BEST BETS:

tops
DOS: Slim-fitting menswear shirts with hems at the hipbone; wrist-length, slim-fitting Empires; V-necks, scoop-necks or boatnecks; textured turtlenecks that aren't skin tight.
DON'TS: Any top that hits at your waist, thus spotlighting what's below.

coats
DOS: Princess; single-breasted; A-line.
DON'TS: Waist-length puffer.

skirts
DOS: Knee-length A-lines are best. A flared hem makes round hips seem narrower in comparison.
DON'TS: Clingy or super-full, with not-stitched-down pleats.

pants
DOS: Choose lowish-rise, flat-front boot-cut pants and jeans. Buy to fit through the hips—the waist can be taken in by a tailor.
DON'TS: Drawstring'd; gathered; pleated, cuffed or tapered ankles—emphasizing skinny ankles makes what's above look wider.

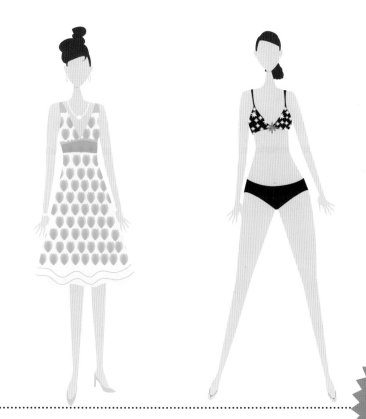

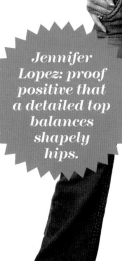

AT NIGHT

- Choose Empire-waisted dresses in flowy fabrics to skim and smooth your silhouette.

- Yes to V-necks! They're torso-lengthening.

- A wide collar (on anything) gives a horizontal emphasis that helps balance you out.

AT THE BEACH

- Keep the focus on top with bright patterns or details like ruffles or shirring.

- Wide-set straps help broaden shoulders to keep you in proportion.

- Dark bottoms with a slightly high-cut leg help downplay hips and thighs, while lengthening legs.

dresses

DOS: Flowy-fabric Empire waist with A-line skirts; wide-set straps; A-line sheaths; knee length.
DON'TS: Clingy, overly full-skirted.

swimsuits

DOS: Minimizer one-pieces with 18-plus percent spandex; bikinis or one-pieces with wide-set straps or V-neck; brighter top, darker bottom. (Tankinis are genius.)
DON'TS: Boy-leg styles or super-high-cut legs.

style tips

- *Avoid outfits that cut you in half at the waist. Highlighting that dividing line makes your lower half look bigger.*

- *Wear dark colors below your waist or one color from head to toe.*

- *Look for a sleek torso-fit jacket with a hipbone or fingertip length. Avoid ones that cover just to the thigh—they draw attention.*

- *Tie on a scarf, layer long necklaces or otherwise play up your upper half.*

IF YOU'RE CURVY...

YOU *have*
A full bust and hips—and, possibly, a dress size of 14 or bigger.

YOU *want*
To minimize curves but not deny they're there.

YOUR *challenge*
Finding clothes that fit—that you love. They're out there!

ARE YOU CURVY *and* **PETITE?**
Cuffed pants make you look shorter.

Blazers should be fitted and hit at your hipbone.

Skirts longer than mid-knee overwhelm you.

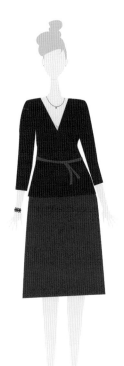

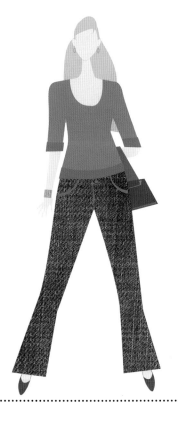

AT WORK
- An open neckline flatters your bust.
- The best tops and jackets are hipbone or wrist length, not shorter or longer.
- Look for fabrics that drape over curves.
- An A-line or not-skin-tight pencil skirt balances your top and bottom.

ON THE WEEKEND
- A scoop-neck fitted tee shows shape without revealing too much.
- Bootcut jeans help balance your hips.
- Low or mid-heels (not high ones for a look this casual) lengthen legs, and you.

YOUR BEST BETS:

tops
DOS: V-necks, or scoop-necks or boatnecks that fit relatively close or, if loose, can be belted at the waist (like a draw-neck gypsy look); halters. Single-breasted jackets.
DON'TS: Gaping between buttons. Big lapels, which draw eyes to your chest.

coats
DOS: Waist-aware styles: princess; single-breasted, belted trench.
DON'TS: Waist-length puffer.

skirts
DOS: Pencil with a slight taper at the knee; A-line; bias cuts; stitch-down pleats.
DON'TS: Fitted at the waist, then full.

pants
DOS: On-the-hip flat-fronts; subtly flared cuffs, because if you're proportioned and tallish, cuffs are fine; straight-leg or boot-cut pants and jeans; straight (not tapered or flared) capris.
DON'TS: Pleated and/or ankle-tapered pants.

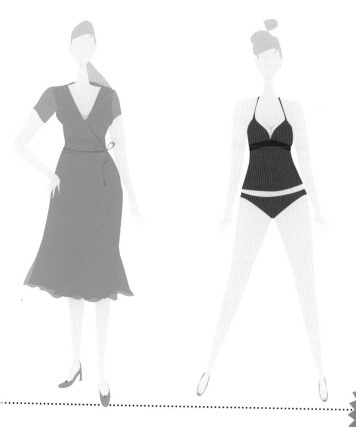

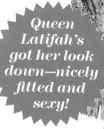

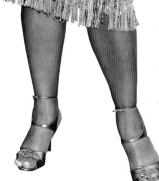

Queen Latifah's got her look down—nicely fitted and sexy!

AT NIGHT

- A wrap dress adjusts to tailor-fit *your* hourglass.

- A narrow or self-tie belt is best.

- Fabrics with a bit of structure skim your curves without hugging them.

- A *small*-scale allover pattern can brilliantly flatter curves.

AT THE BEACH

- Hip-riding briefs are all-around flattering—much more so than those old-fashioned "skirted" bottoms.

- Lots of spandex (18-plus percent) delivers support and control.

- Halter tops are great for customized support, but if you find they pull on your neck, opt for an x-back top—comfort *and* lift.

dresses

DOS: Wraps; princess-shapes; sheaths; sundresses.
DON'TS: Fifties-style full-skirt dresses in a big-scale pattern. Tight satin dresses.

swimsuits

DOS: Bra-cuts; halters; long-top tankinis; on-the-hip briefs; unflimsy bikinis with bust support; 18-plus percent spandex for control and support.
DON'TS: Granny-style skirt suits, baggy fabrics.

style tips

- Aim for a silhouette where one piece (top or bottom) is loose-fitting, the other closer-fitting.

- Dress head to toe in one color or shades of one color.

- Get properly fitted bras—you need the right coverage and support to look great in clothes!

- Try on tees before you buy and avoid ones that ride up in front.

IF YOU'RE
BOY-SHAPED...

YOU
have
A straight shape, up and down: narrow hips, small bust and not-so-curvy waist.

YOU
want
To look like you've got curves (without surgical intervention).

YOUR
challenge
To add visual details that create a womanly shape.

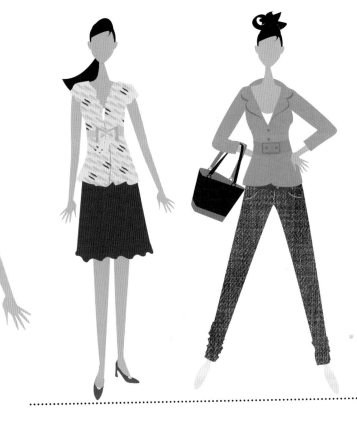

AT WORK

- A ruffled shirt and nipped waist are curve-builders on top.

- Skirts with a little swing are good for you—they create hips better than, say, a boxy mini.

ON THE WEEKEND

- Lucky you! Just about any jeans look great on slim hips.

- A tailored, curvy jacket (not boy-cut) gives you a feminine shape.

YOUR BEST BETS:

tops
DOS: Halters, cap-sleeve styles; blouson tops with ribbed or banded hems that hit at the wide part of your hips; nipped-waist tailored jackets.
DON'TS: Tight V-necks. Plain camisoles or tanks unless they're layered under another piece.

coats
DOS: Princess; double-breasted; belted; ribbed-at-the-hip or longer; shapely puffers.
DON'TS: Oversized anything.

skirts
DOS: Pleated, trumpet, flared hem, A-line, pouf, pegged. The inherent femininity of skirts works wonders. Shorter hemlines make you look curvier.
DON'TS: Straight-cut minis (picture a square of fabric)—they won't add curves.

pants
DOS: Skinny *or* slightly flared; low-waist *or* high-waist cuts.
DON'TS: Very full or baggy.

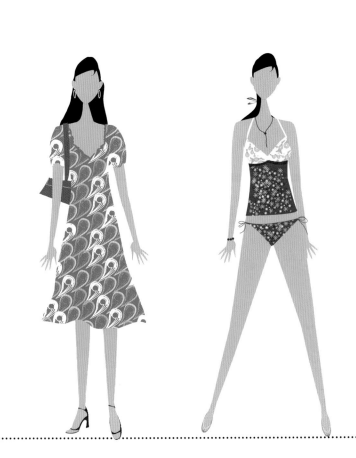

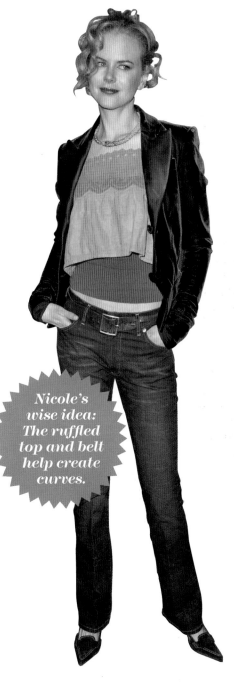

AT NIGHT

- Make a swingy, bias-cut dress even sexier with girly heels.

- A neckline that accentuates your bust (vs., say, a strapless cut that flattens it) looks good on you.

- Fuller sleeves and floaty fabrics are also smart buys for you.

AT THE BEACH

- A halter top can make more of a small chest. Ruffles help, too.

- Highlight your waist or bust with a contrasting color or other detail.

- Side ties can add a smidge to your hips.

- Low-slung bottoms with a high-cut leg make you look more hourglassy.

dresses

DOS: Angled seams and bias cuts that create curves; halters; anything with details at your waist.
DON'TS: Snug knits.

swimsuits

DOS: Prints, small ruffles, details that accent curves.
DON'TS: Plain black one-piece.

style tips

- Avoid clothes that mimic your straight lines—formless skirts, boxy jackets and tunics, blah sheath dresses.

- Wear off-the-body cuts, and nip your waist with a belt to fake a curvier silhouette.

- Go for detail or texture (gathering, shirring) at your bustline. Horizontal-stripe tees were made for you.

- Use layers to build curves, like a flowy blouse beneath a cardigan or wrap sweater (let the blouse hem flirt below the sweater hem), or a fitted tee under a thin-strap Empire top or dress.

IF YOU'RE
PETITE...

YOU
have
A proportioned body, with a height of 5'3" or under.

YOU
want
To dress with the same grown-up sophistication, sexiness and authority that your 5'7" friends do.

YOUR
challenge
Zeroing in on the pieces and combinations that elevate your look.

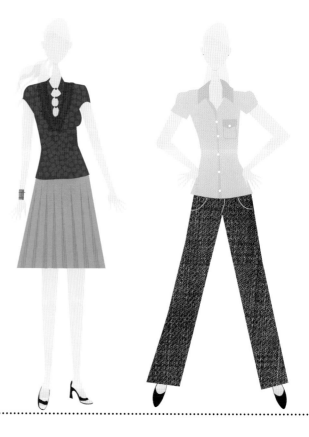

AT WORK

- A-line or pencil skirts are universally flattering.

- Your best hemline is a little *above* the knee, to lengthen legs.

- A hip-length top is torso-lengthening.

- Open-toe shoes can elongate. Pass on all ankle-strap styles, though.

ON THE WEEKEND

- Long, low-rise jeans work for you, but they shouldn't be so low that they make a horizontal line across the widest part of your hips.

- Snug-fitting tops that show off your womanly shape are better than shapeless ones that'll swallow you.

YOUR BEST BETS:

tops
DOS: Belted wraps; floaty, just-past-your-waist looks; fitted blazers; V- and scoop-necks.
DON'TS: Oversized tops.

coats
DOS: Princess; single-breasted; belted; midthigh puffers.
DON'TS: Swing coats.

skirts
DOS: A-line; stitch-down pleats; pencil; knee-length.
DON'TS: Full; too-long.

pants
DOS: Low-waisted; close-fitting through waist and hips; straight or subtly boot-cut. Hems that hit the middle of your bare heel.
DON'TS: Wide; cuffed.

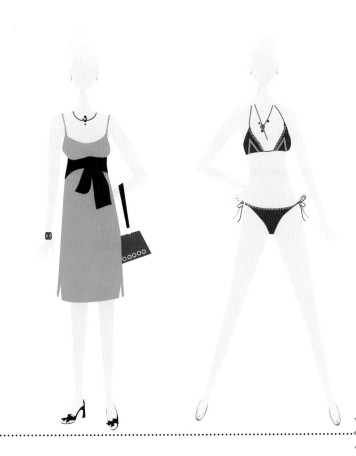

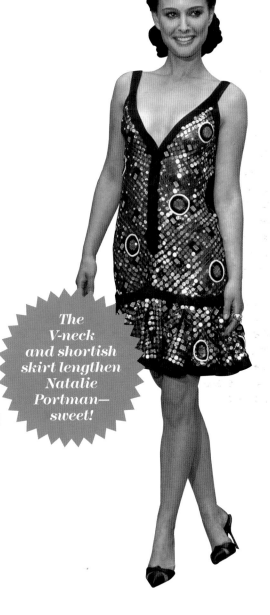

The V-neck and shortish skirt lengthen Natalie Portman— sweet!

AT NIGHT

- A V-neckline is always a height-enhancing detail.

- A sleek-fitting, top-of-the-knee Empire dress appears to lengthen you.

- An embellished bustline draws the eye up.

- Pointy-toe heels elongate legs.

AT THE BEACH

- Show your curves! Who'll notice your height?

- A halter brings eyes up and plays up your bust.

- Highish-cut legs are excellent lengtheners.

dresses

DOS: Sheaths; shirtdresses with floaty, not full, skirts; Empires.
DON'TS: Trapezes; long and blousy.

swimsuits

DOS: Allover pattern string bikinis, as bare as you want to go; V-neck one-pieces; side cut-out one-piece.
DON'TS: Thinking that height matters in a swimsuit!

style tips

- *Learn which brands run small (hint: most European ones) and buy them religiously.*

- *Wear one color head to toe: It adds instant height.*

- *Find a tailor you love. He or she will be that important in your life.*

- *Try tops that come to your hipbone, skimming past your waist, with a slender skirt or pants.*

- *A two-inch heel is your all-purpose ideal.*

IF YOU'RE
BUSTY...

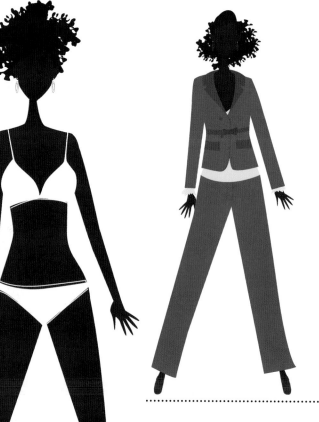

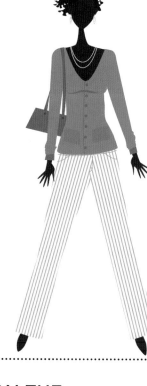

YOU
have
What thousands of women pay boatloads of cash for: a more-than-generous bustline.

YOU
want
To A) dress so that your breasts aren't the first thing people notice about you; and B) look evenly pro-portioned.

YOUR
challenge
To show (as in, not hide) your bustline, without flaunting it.

AT WORK
- Feminine figures look fantastic in mens-wear-style pieces like a pantsuit.
- V-, scoop- and other open necklines work for you—just don't go *too* bare.
- Pants with a bit of flare help balance your top and bottom proportions.

ON THE WEEKEND
- A fitted—not tight—sweater looks chic.
- Dark on top and lighter shades below will bal-ance your silhouette.
- Boot-cut jeans are for you. Super-flared legs, in jeans or pants, are less flattering.

YOUR BEST BETS:

tops
DOS: Fairly fitted V- or scoop-necklines. Tops that taper or nip your waist a bit.
DON'TS: Droopy blousons. Empire waists, which are like shining a spotlight on your breasts. Straps that don't cover your bra's.

coats
DOS: Princess; single-breasted, belted; knee-length puffers.
DON'TS: Waist-length puffers.

skirts
DOS: A-line; pencil when it's paired with a tailored jacket; stitch-down pleats; knee lengths.
DON'TS: Midthigh and narrow. They'll make you look top-heavy.

pants
DOS: Subtle flares; lowish-waisted.
DON'TS: Extremely skinny *or* full.

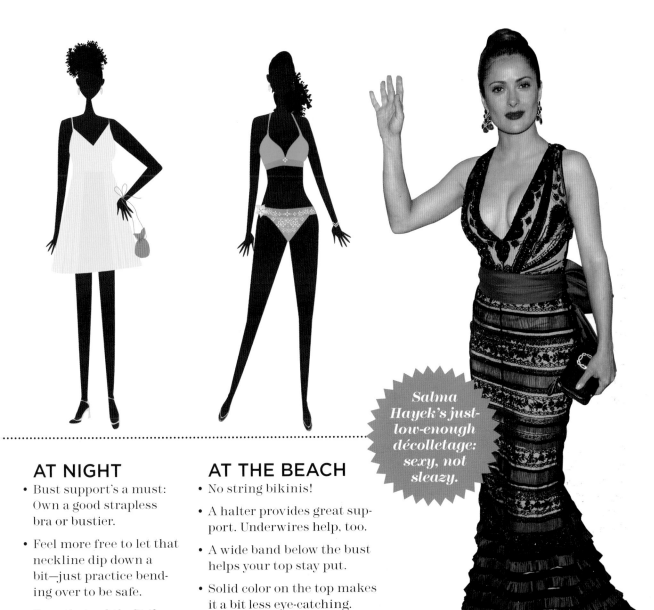

Salma Hayek's just-low-enough décolletage: sexy, not sleazy.

AT NIGHT

- Bust support's a must: Own a good strapless bra or bustier.

- Feel more free to let that neckline dip down a bit—just practice bending over to be safe.

- Tops that subtly fit the torso and waist, with flirty flow below, are better than allover loose.

AT THE BEACH

- No string bikinis!

- A halter provides great support. Underwires help, too.

- A wide band below the bust helps your top stay put.

- Solid color on the top makes it a bit less eye-catching.

- The coverage on the bottom should be in proportion to the top, not teensy-weensy.

dresses

DOS: Controlled on top, a little fuller below the waist. Body-skimming sheath dresses look amazing on you.
DON'TS: Full on top and bottom *and* belted.

swimsuits

DOS: Bikinis or low-neck, highish-leg one-pieces; underwires and/or substantial halters (not string).
DON'TS: All-cotton triangle bikinis.

style tips

- *Steer clear of big patterns, ruffles, embroidery or other attention-grabbing details on top.*

- *Get fitted for a bra by a true pro, at a department store or boutique. Everything will look, feel and fit better when you're in the right bra. (P.S. minimizers work.)*

- *Favor fabrics with body (like crisp, woven cotton), not flimsy ones, on top.*

- *Benefit from spandex. A little stretch gives the controlled look and fit you want.*

WHAT TO WEAR
UNDER THERE

YOUR *essential* BOTTOMS

There's some flexibility here. If you can't abide thongs, for example, skip 'em. As with bras, seamless, silky and stretchy fabrics are best for a no-show and no-cling look. (All-cotton's trickier.)

....

how to avoid VPL forever

- DO wear plain, seamless nylon hipster or bikini briefs that fit well under your butt.

- DO try silky boy shorts instead of a thong with flowy skirts and dresses.

- DO wear a thong/brief hybrid (totally bare in back, brieflike waist and sides).

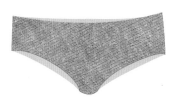

LOW-RISE BRIEF
These should hug right under your butt for a smooth line under clothes.

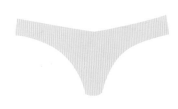

LOW-RISE THONG
Some uncomfortable thongs will make you feel like you have a permanent wedgie, so shop around until you find one you can wear all day.

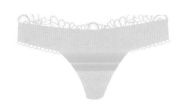

SEXY LITTLE SOMETHING
Match these to your sexy little bra.

PLUS OTHER USEFUL BOTTOMS TO OWN
Boy shorts
Black sheer pantyhose
Silky half-slip
Black opaque hose or tights

LOOK SLIMMER INSTANTLY (HONEST!)
Celebs' body-flattery secret weapon can be yours, too, with shapewear—lingerie that slims. Pick from a range of pieces to get one that whittles the zone you're targeting, and from a range of control levels: light (around 15 percent spandex, like control-top hose); moderate (15 to 30 percent, adds more control); or firm (35 percent or more, vaporizes inches but may feel uncomfortable after a few hours). Herroom.com and barenecessities.com are good sources.

YOUR
essential
BRAS

Build your bra wardrobe on these four basic styles, and make sure to have the ones you wear most often in a skin-matching color.

....

how to tell if your bra really fits

THE FIT'S A DO IF:

- you've been measured by a pro within the past year
- the center of the bra sits flat against your sternum
- it doesn't roam when you make arm circles
- your breasts look perky, not saggy
- it passes the tell-all tight white tee test
- you're pretty much unaware of it all day

THE FIT'S A DON'T IF:

- you assumed that if you're a 34B, that a 36A would fit
- the underwires cut into your breasts at the sides, instead of cupping around them
- the back sits higher than the base of your shoulder blades
- the cups crinkle or gap

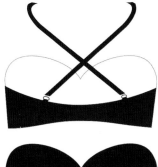

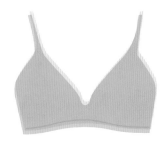

CONVERTIBLE BRA
Can be worn strapless, racerback or as a halter-top; a must for bare looks.

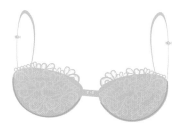

EVERYDAY BRA
Molded cup, soft cup, seamless stretch and demi are all good options.

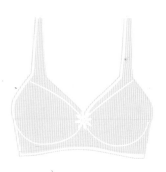

SEXY LITTLE BRA
The aphrodisiac of your collection—think bare and lacy in a gorgeous color.

MINIMIZING OR ENHANCING BRA
Go up or down about one cup size with one of these (and sure, make one your everyday bra if you like).

....

PLUS OTHER USEFUL BRAS AND LINGERIE TOPS TO OWN

T-shirt bra in a skin-matching shade to wear under white tees

Stretchy camisole with built-in bra

Silky, lacy camisole

Adhesive "stick-on bra" for under the most plunging or backless tops (try victoriassecret.com or figleaves.com)

DON'T give your thong the spotlight.

You need a full-coverage bra—otherwise, it's a **DON'T**.

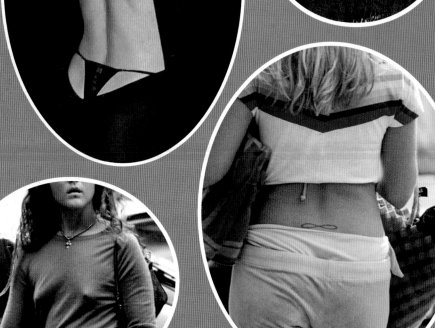

No matter your cup size, the no-bra look is a **DON'T**.

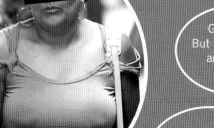

Great body! But visible undies are always a **DON'T**.

We **DON'T** need to see every detail—a strapless bra would solve this.

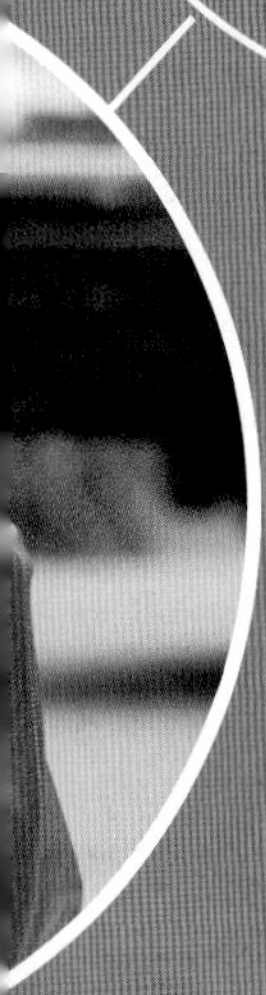

DON'T let your undies creep up on you—OUCH!

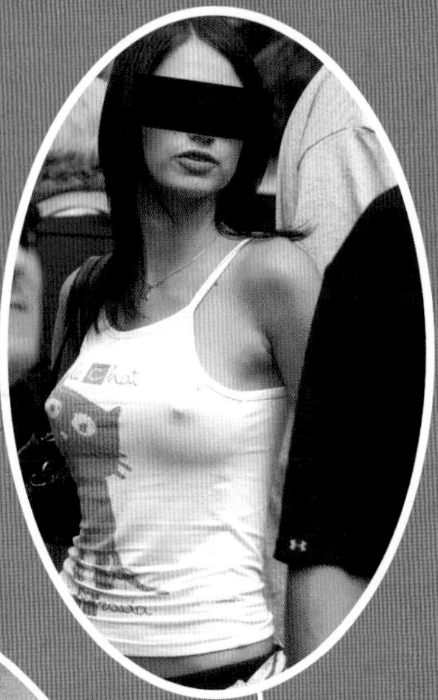

They may be perky, but it's still a ***DON'T.***

Tight bra under tight shirt? It's a ***DON'T***.

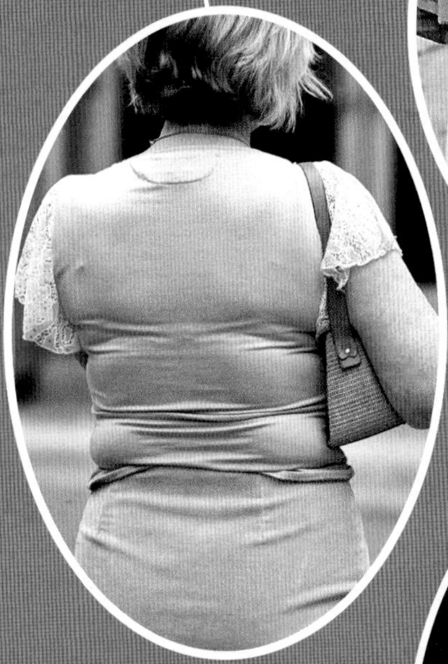

DON'T wear lumpy undies under tight white pants.

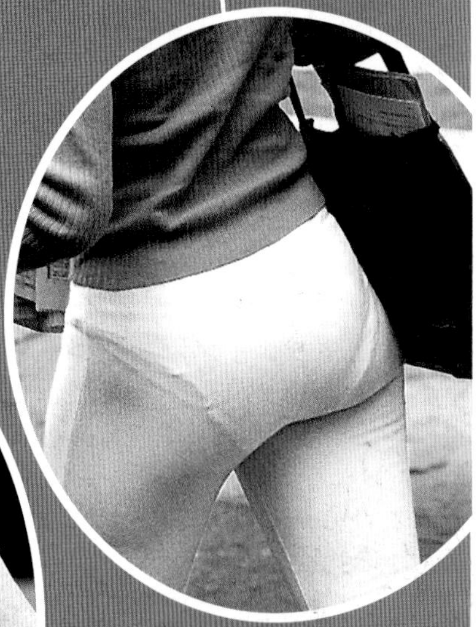

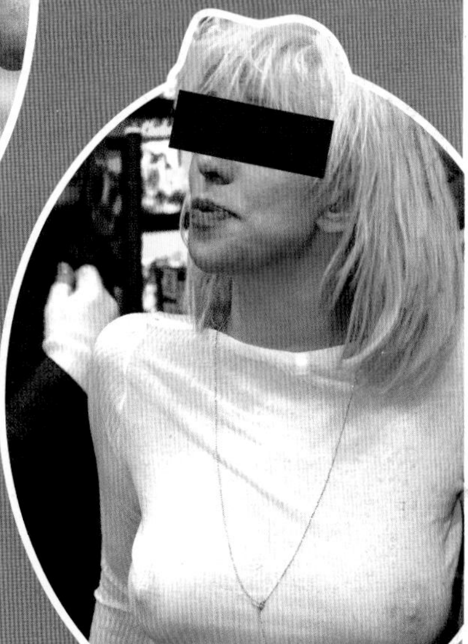

DON'T go braless under a see-through top.

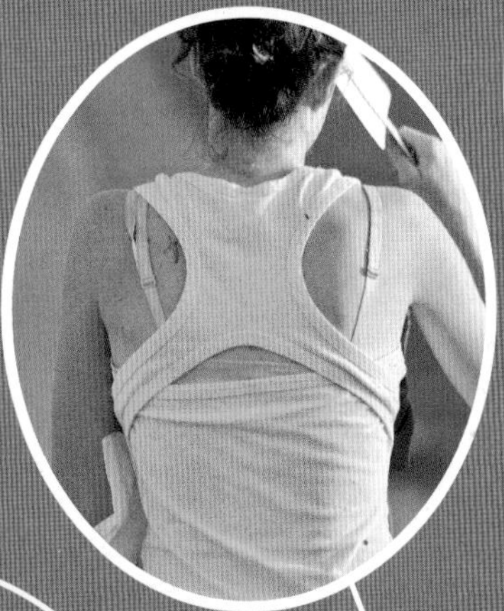

We know it's trendy, but ***DON'T*** take the visible bra thing this far.

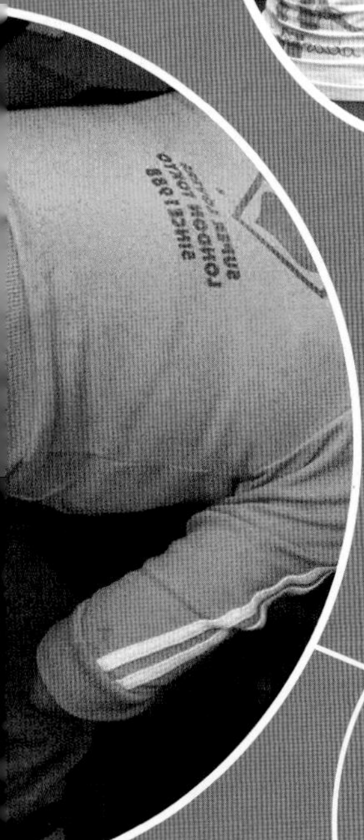

The only way to avoid this ***DON'T?*** Buy higher-waisted pants!

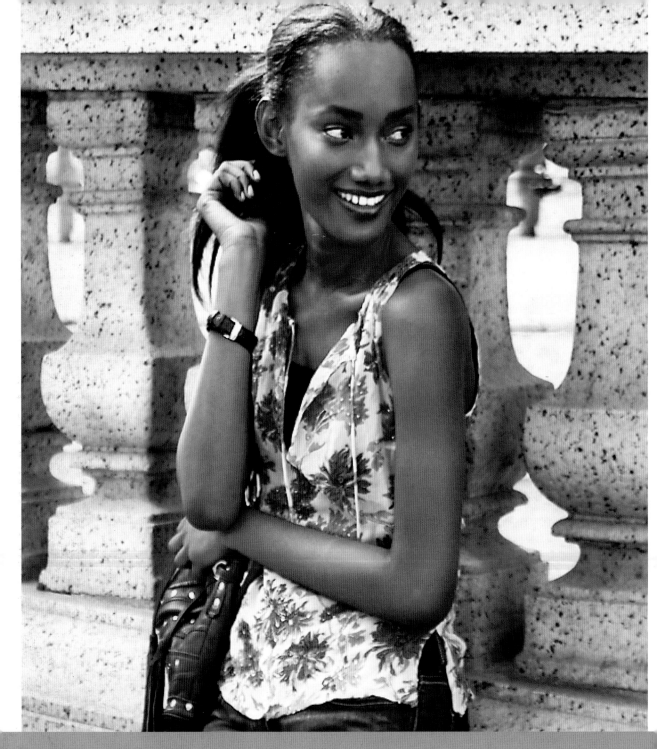

YOUR

DO

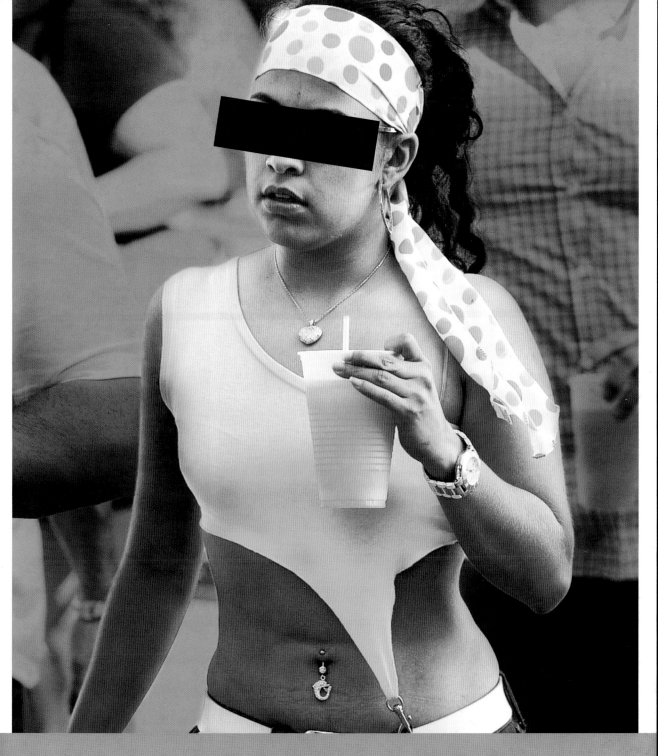

WEEKEND LIFE

WHAT WORKS—AND WHAT DOESN'T—
IN YOUR DOWNTIME

DON'T

THE RULES
for weekends

(1)

TREAT SATURDAY AND SUNDAY AS A TIME FOR STYLE EXPERIMENTING.

Seize the weekend to try out trickier stuff, like crazy vintage accessories or super-high heels—without getting funny looks from your coworkers.

(2)

PLAY WITH YOUR HAIR, TOO.

Try accessories, braids, new products or even an elaborate updo, embarrassment-free.

(3)

HAVE AT LEAST THREE WHITE T-SHIRTS THAT FIT AND FEEL GREAT.

Wear them alone on weekends or layered under everything all year long.

(4)

INVEST IN A FITTED, FINE-KNIT CARDIGAN IN YOUR FAVORITE COLOR.

It's an easy way to tie together casual pieces.

RESTRICT "HOUSE CLOTHES"—RATTY SWEATS, FADED SHIRTS, HOLEY SOCKS—TO THE HOUSE.

Even if you're just bound for the cleaners, throw on jeans and a clean shirt instead. And a bra, too. It won't kill you. What if you run into your mother? Or ex?

SWITCH TO A WEEKEND-SPECIFIC BAG.

You wouldn't wear work pumps with shorts and a tee, right? Your bag's mood should match your look.

BRING OUT YOUR BROKEN-IN—BUT NOT RIPPED-UP—JEANS.

Faded is fine, but tatters and tears should be minimal unless you're painting the house or digging in the garden.

IF YOU CAN FOLLOW ONLY ONE RULE, THIS IS IT!

STAY TRUE TO WHAT FITS YOUR BODY.

Weekend dressing is relaxed, but you should still stick with the shapes and styles that flatter your figure best. Experiment with trends and sexy pieces—just the ones that look good on you.

KEEP YOUR TOES PRETTY.

Live in flip-flops? Expose your feet to the world only after you've given them TLC.

WEAR YOUR COMFORT-ZONE SWIMSUIT.

Skimpy, flashy, sporty, tame— buy the suit only if you'll enjoy being bare in it.

TOPS

THE BEST WEEKEND TOPS

You want shirts that are comfy, but they don't have to be shapeless. Search for body-skimming styles in casual fabrics: Super-baggy shapes are too hard to wear.

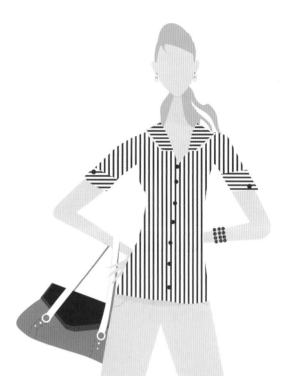

① BUTTON-DOWN

- Choose this tailored style when you want to look put-together.
- Go for casual fabrics like linen and cotton. (In silk, this style looks office-y.)
- If you have a favorite oversize shirt, just add a sweet tank or a belt to give it style.
- Three-quarter-length sleeves are a feminine touch, but good old rolled-up cuffs work too!

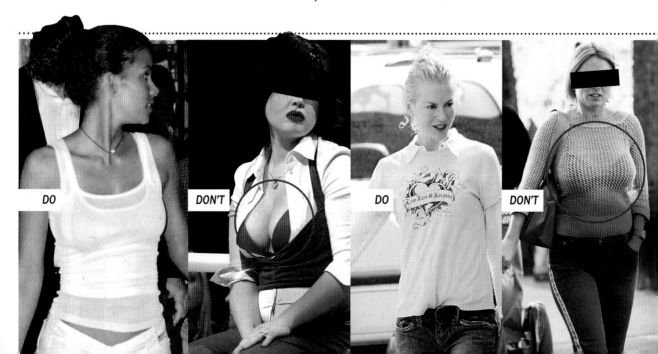

DO

DON'T

DO

DON'T

TANK

- Pick wider straps that cover your bra completely.

- Steer clear of ultra-sheer knits, which cling to every ripple.

- Men's ribbed T-shirts are long, but that's where their virtues end. Opt for made-for-women styles that fit femininely under a jacket, sweater or button-down.

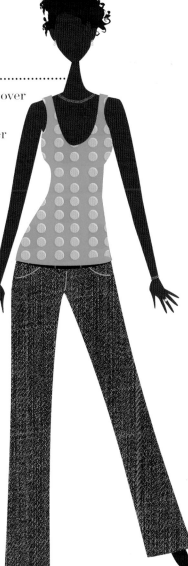

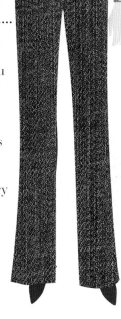

T-SHIRT

- Go for fitted styles, but avoid anything too tight or short—you want it to hit roughly at your hips.

- Your shirt's most important feature: its neckline. Find the shape that's best on you and buy it in every color under the sun.

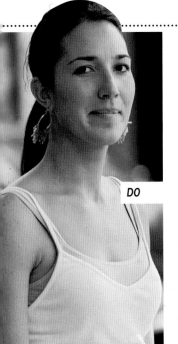

DO

Style Clinic

Layered tops: how to be a DO

Layerable T-shirts are the basis of a weekend wardrobe. Thick, boxy ones cause unsightly bunching, so look for close-fitting, lightweight cotton styles instead. This brings us to a common DON'T: If you can see through your tee, wear it over something more substantial.

"Layering is a great way to play with fashion and color. You can look edgy with a short-sleeve tee over a long-sleeve shirt, or pretty with a tank peeking out under a scoopneck."
—CLAIRE STANSFIELD, C & C CALIFORNIA DESIGNER

THE BIG
DOS&DON'TS OF
TOPS

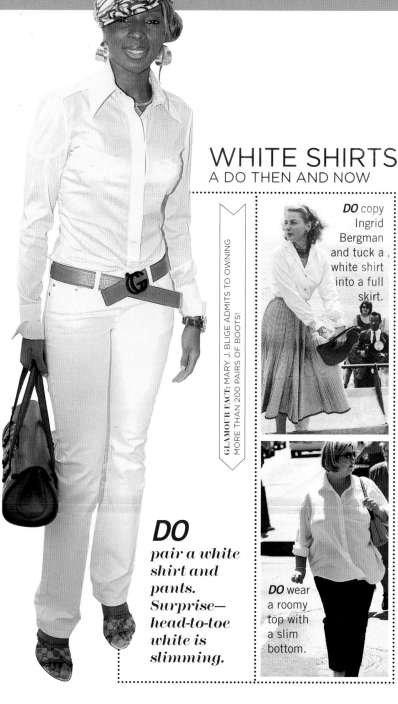

WHITE SHIRTS
A DO THEN AND NOW

GLAMOUR FACT: MARY J. BLIGE ADMITS TO OWNING MORE THAN 200 PAIRS OF BOOTS!

DO copy Ingrid Bergman and tuck a white shirt into a full skirt.

DO
pair a white shirt and pants. Surprise— head-to-toe white is slimming.

DO wear a roomy top with a slim bottom.

GET
SUPPORT
WE ALL NEED IT!

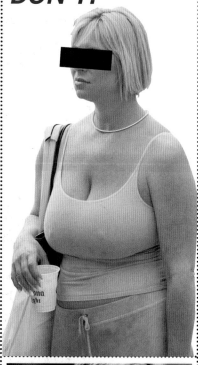

Ouch! This just looks painful.
DON'T!

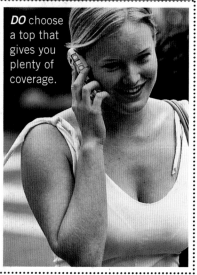

DO choose a top that gives you plenty of coverage.

TOPS ON
THE LOOSE!

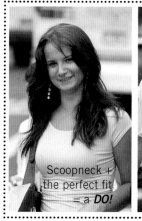

Scoopneck + the perfect fit = a **DO!**

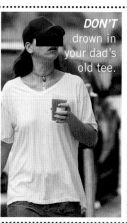

DON'T drown in your dad's old tee.

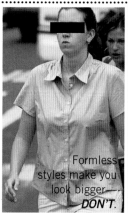

Formless styles make you look bigger— **DON'T.**

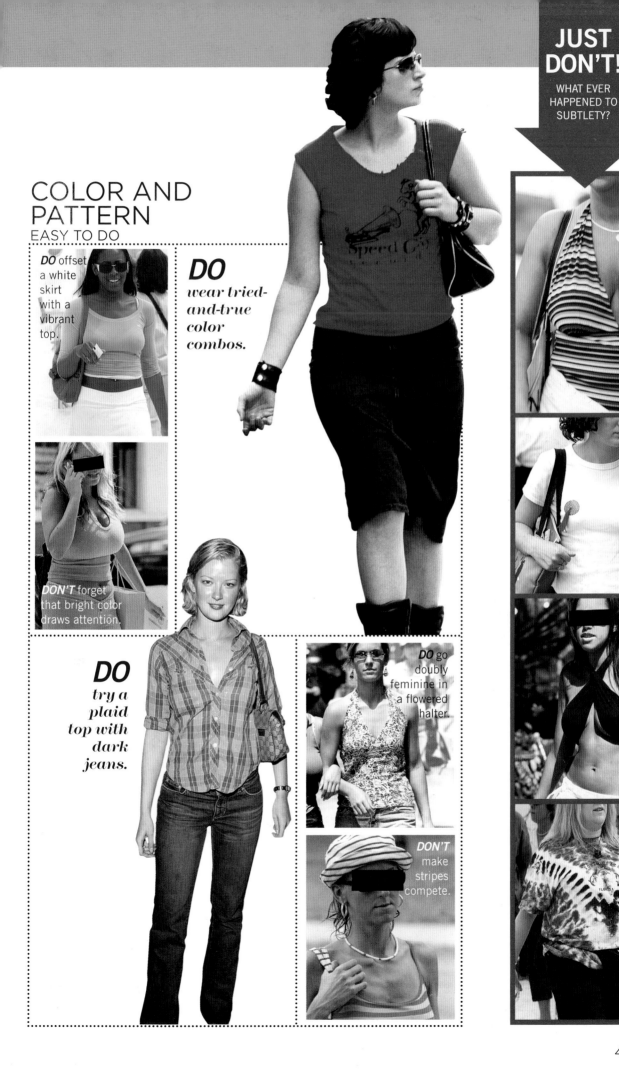

COLOR AND PATTERN
EASY TO DO

DO offset a white skirt with a vibrant top.

DON'T forget that bright color draws attention.

DO
wear tried-and-true color combos.

DO
try a plaid top with dark jeans.

DO go doubly feminine in a flowered halter.

DON'T make stripes compete.

41

DENIM

THREE WAYS TO WEAR DENIM ON THE WEEKEND

Chances are, you wear denim all weekend long. Who doesn't? No matter the item, color or length you love, beware these universal DON'Ts: excessive bleaching and inconsistent coloring, rips and holes and embellishment overload. Oh, and pleats.

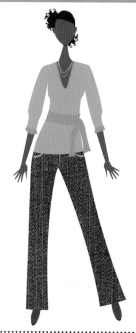

JEANS

- Prepare yourself to try on at least five or six pairs. Each brand's fit and sizing vary, and some are cut with only particular body types in mind (sadly!).

- Bend over, squat and check the back view before you buy!

- A subtle boot cut in a dark color is the most flattering jean on every body type.

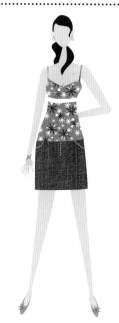

JEANS SKIRT

- Look for a style that sits low on your hips; it elongates a short torso.

- Make sure you can bend over without exposing your underwear or yourself!

- Pair with ballet flats for a girly twist.

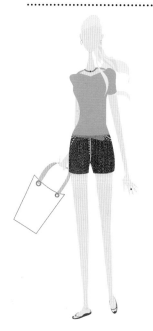

JEANS SHORTS

- Don't go shorter than midthigh. Too long *always* beats too short.

- Skip faded, whiskered styles and opt for a single-color wash.

- Finish with flat sandals or flip-flops—never heels!

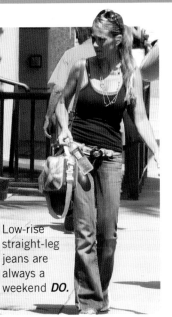

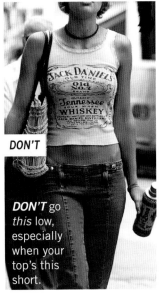

DON'T

DO tuck skinny jeans into boots for a long-legged look.

Low-rise straight-leg jeans are always a weekend **DO**.

DON'T go *this* low, especially when your top's this short.

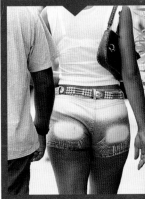

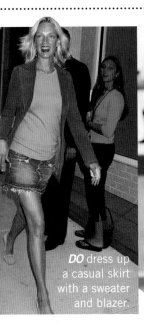

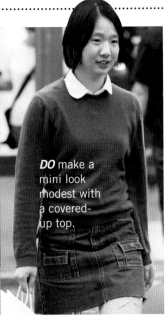

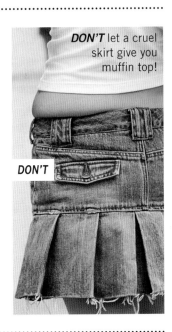

DON'T let a cruel skirt give you muffin top!

DO make a mini look modest with a covered-up top.

DON'T

DO dress up a casual skirt with a sweater and blazer.

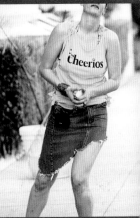

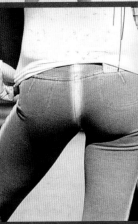

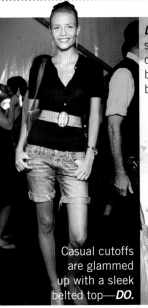

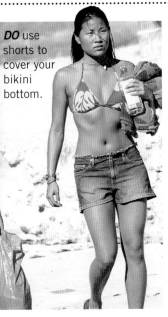

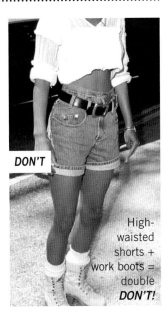

DO use shorts to cover your bikini bottom.

DON'T

Casual cutoffs are glammed up with a sleek belted top—**DO**.

High-waisted shorts + work boots = double **DON'T!**

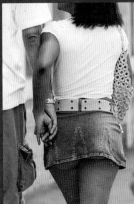

43

PANTS & SHORTS

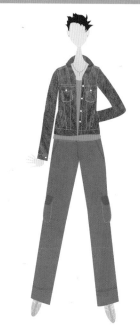

① CARGO PANTS

- Don't use government-issue fatigues as inspiration: Actual camouflage is hard to pull off.

- Keep 'em looking feminine by pairing with a formfitting top.

- Add an open, sexy shoe like sandals, wedges or flats.

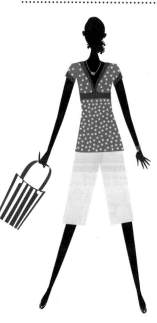

② LONG SHORTS

- Look for a straight-cut knee-skimming length that works on every body type.

- Opt for a neutral, solid color for maximum versatility.

- Pair with sandals or flats—no workout sneakers!

WAIT! INSTEAD OF JEANS, WEAR *THESE*

The three alternative bottoms here are as good-looking and wearable as your favorite blues. Shorts, no longer the fear-inducing relic from the '70s, come in lots of lengths and fits now. And cargo pants will take you everywhere you need to go—but for flattery's sake, don't overstuff the pockets!

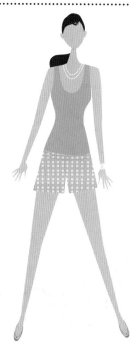

③ SHORT SHORTS

- Remember, "short" is relative. Even on the weekend, there's such a thing as showing too much skin.

- Balance them out with a substantial top, like a peasant blouse, tunic or long tee or tank.

- Pair with flats, sandals or wedges—stilettos look too vampy.

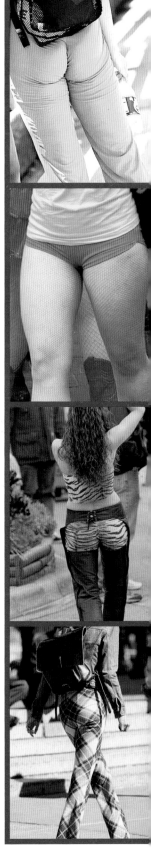

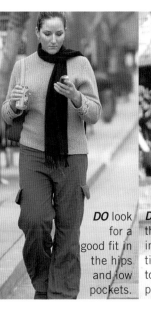

DO look for a good fit in the hips and low pockets.

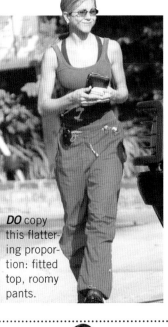

DO copy this flattering proportion: fitted top, roomy pants.

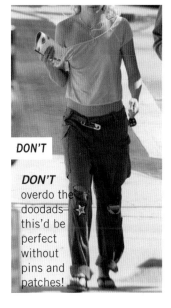

DON'T

DON'T overdo the doodads—this'd be perfect without pins and patches!

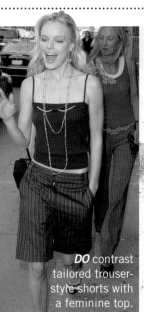

DO contrast tailored trouser-style shorts with a feminine top.

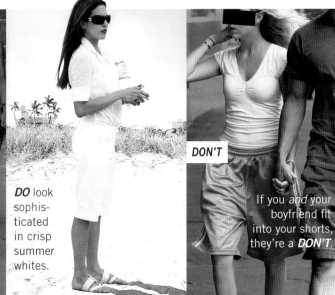

DO look sophisticated in crisp summer whites.

DON'T

If you *and* your boyfriend fit into your shorts, they're a **DON'T**.

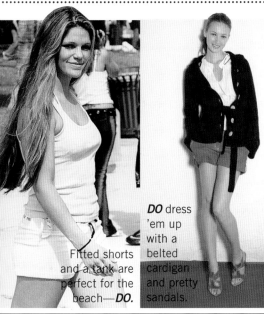

Fitted shorts and a tank are perfect for the beach—**DO.**

DO dress 'em up with a belted cardigan and pretty sandals.

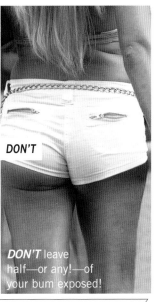

DON'T

DON'T leave half—or any!—of your bum exposed!

GLAMOUR FACT: BECAUSE THE SHORTS WORN BY CATHERINE BACH AS DAISY DUKE ON TV'S *THE DUKES OF HAZZARD* WERE THOUGHT TO BE TOO REVEALING, SHE WORE PANTYHOSE UNDERNEATH.

45

SWEATERS

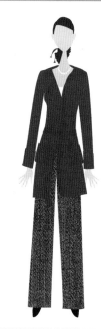

1

SWEATER JACKET

- Add a belt to give your waist instant definition.

- Make sure that yours hits at your knee or above— any longer and it looks like a pricey bathrobe.

- Pair with slim pants. A very full pant or skirt makes the look seem dowdy.

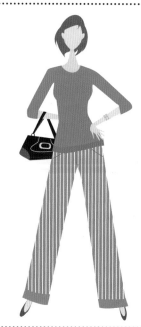

2

CREWNECK

- Opt for body-close styles— not man-cut ones.

- Choose a crewneck with minimal or no ribbing at the hem for the sleekest no-bumps look.

- Add a fitted tee or blouse underneath for a sporty/Frenchy look.

THREE SWEATERS EVERY WOMAN SHOULD OWN

Stock up on sweaters in different styles and weights and you'll wear them year-round. Fine-gauge merino wool, cashmere and cotton are best for bulk-free layering.

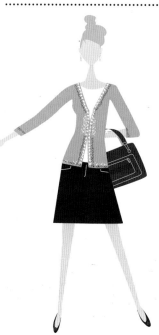

3

EMBELLISHED CARDIGAN

- Go for small beads or embroidery—more versatile than mega-decoration.

- Grab a bright, fun color, with a slim, ladylike fit.

- Mix this staple with everything. Wear it over a Saturday-night cocktail dress or Sunday-brunch jeans.

46

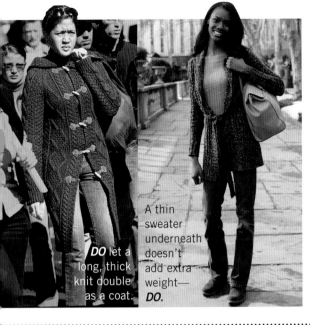

DO let a long, thick knit double as a coat.

A thin sweater underneath doesn't add extra weight— **DO.**

DON'T

DON'T wear a street sweeper!

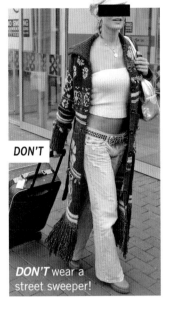

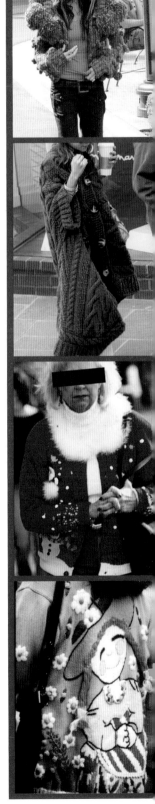

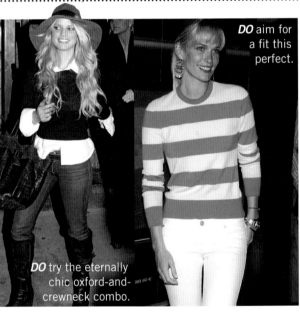

DO try the eternally chic oxford-and-crewneck combo.

DO aim for a fit this perfect.

DON'T

DON'T wear an extra-long sweater with an extra-short skirt.

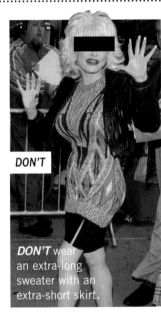

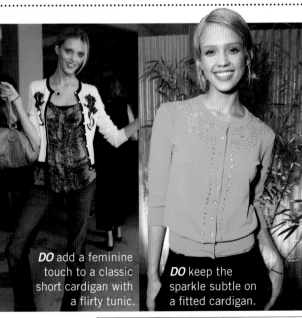

DO add a feminine touch to a classic short cardigan with a flirty tunic.

DO keep the sparkle subtle on a fitted cardigan.

DON'T mix motifs: Oversize floral knits clash with leopard.

DON'T

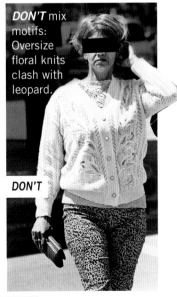

GLAMOUR FACT: JESSICA ALBA'S FAVORITE COLORS ARE PINK AND PURPLE.

47

COATS

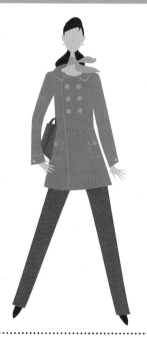

PEACOAT

- Choose a length that hits above the knee. Anything lower ruins the preppy-sportiness of this style.

- If your wardrobe's mostly neutral, pick a bright peacoat. Closet full of colors and prints? Stick with classic navy.

- This double-breasted (meaning double-buttoned) look is best for small to medium chests.

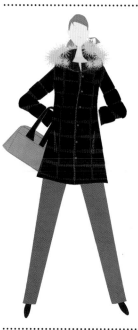

DOWN COAT

- Choose one that nips in a bit at the waist so you don't lose your shape entirely.

- Keep your lower half toasty in a coat that hits midthigh or a jacket that covers your bum.

- Look for armpit vents—a real plus if you'll actually be skiing or sledding in this coat.

THREE CHIC WAYS TO STAY WARM

It's tempting to hunker down inside a giant womb of a coat, but unless it's 50 below, you don't have to abandon style for warmth. Just look for shapes and fabrics, high-tech or natural, that can withstand the elements. Love the quilted look? Go for tailored, not sleeping-baggy. And when you're in the store, try on coats with a sweater to check for wiggle room.

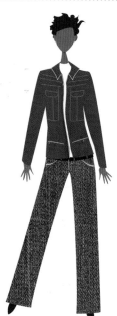

LEATHER JACKET

- With thick material like leather, a jacket is perfect; a trench would be too much.

- Go for unshiny leather; anything that gleams looks cheap.

- Wear yours with denim, a sweater and an attitude.

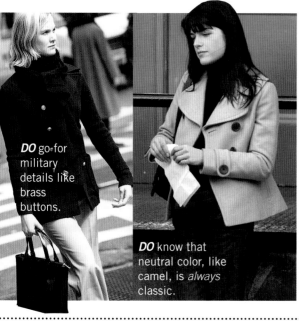

DO go for military details like brass buttons.

DO know that neutral color, like camel, is *always* classic.

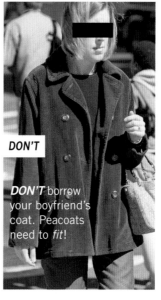

DON'T

DON'T borrow your boyfriend's coat. Peacoats need to *fit*!

JUST DON'T!

SAY NO TO COATS THAT SWALLOW YOUR BODY— AND PRIDE.

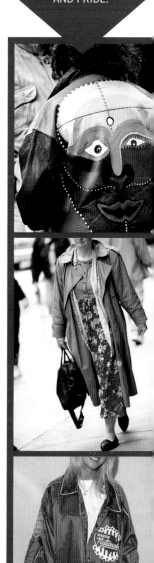

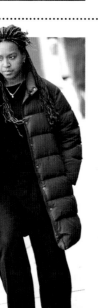

DO keep your snow-white coat squeaky-clean.

DO opt for a dark-color puffer for city chic.

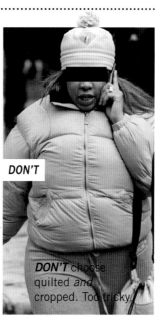

DON'T

DON'T choose quilted *and* cropped. Too tricky.

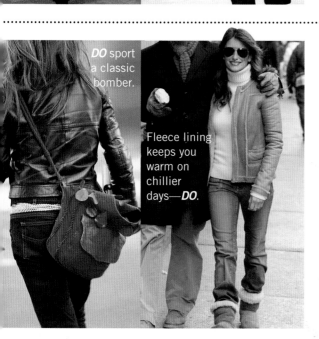

DO sport a classic bomber.

Fleece lining keeps you warm on chillier days—**DO**.

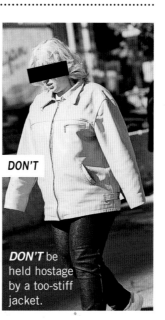

DON'T

DON'T be held hostage by a too-stiff jacket.

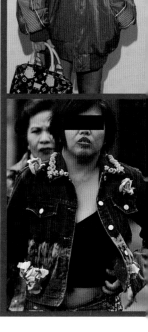

DRESSES & SKIRTS

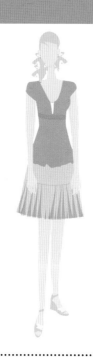

THREE EASY-TO-WEAR STYLES

An airy dress or skirt is a genius way to look great yet still stay casual on the weekends, but beware of shapeless pieces. Don't go too long or too loose or conversely, too short and tight, which will just have you tugging and fidgeting your way through a party. Instead, try a comfortable, body-skimming silhouette in a lightweight fabric.

FLIPPY SKIRT

- Look for lengths that fall slightly above the knee for all-around (front *and* back) flattery.

- Sleekifying detail: no waistband.

- Pair with a snug top for the most body-friendly effect.

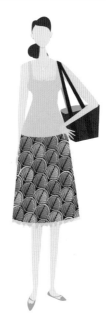

PEASANT SKIRT

- Find one that hits midcalf—anything longer looks sloppy.

- Choose a gently full skirt that rests low—but not too low—on the hips.

- Wear it with kitten-heel sandals or boots and a hip-length, fitted top for an attractive head-to-toe look.

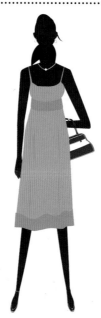

SUNDRESS

- Go for Empire waists; they'll flatter most body types and give you room for dessert.

- Try small, allover prints. They're more minimizing than big florals.

- Throw on a cardigan and flats for a look that'll work all weekend, day to night.

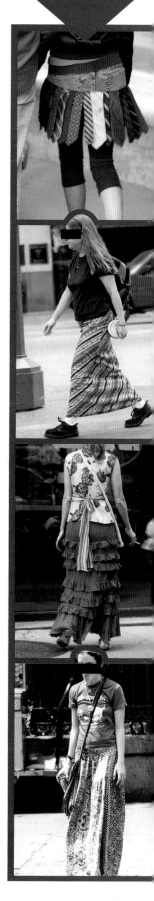

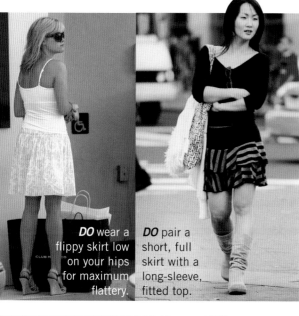

DO wear a flippy skirt low on your hips for maximum flattery.

DO pair a short, full skirt with a long-sleeve, fitted top.

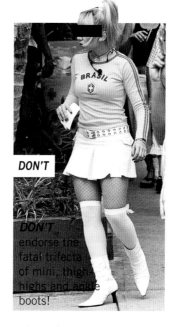

DON'T

DON'T endorse the fatal trifecta of mini, thigh highs and ankle boots!

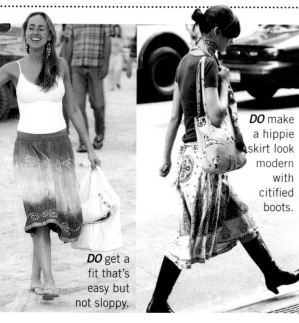

DO get a fit that's easy but not sloppy.

DO make a hippie skirt look modern with citified boots.

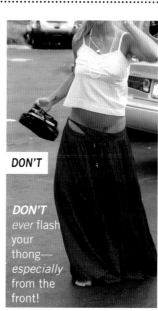

DON'T

DON'T ever flash your thong—*especially* from the front!

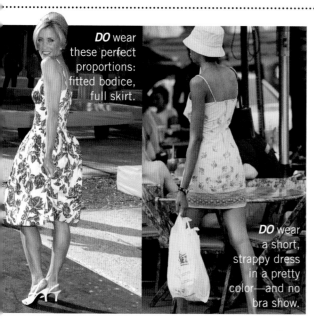

DO wear these perfect proportions: fitted bodice, full skirt.

DO wear a short, strappy dress in a pretty color—and no bra show.

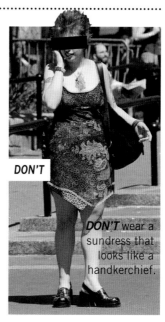

DON'T

DON'T wear a sundress that looks like a handkerchief.

SWIMSUITS

THREE PERFECT SUITS

Okay, so venturing into the fitting room, swimsuits in tow, is one of the most un-fun shopping experiences ever. But remember these foolproof fit rules, and it'll be a lot easier: Most swimsuit DON'Ts result from too little support or too much exposure. Make sure you're well supported on top—a halter with underwire is your safest bet—and adequately covered on bottom. And attention, active types: Even the most secure-seeming bikini bottoms, and tops, fall off, so a one-piece might be *your* best bet.

TWO-PIECE

- Make sure that there's enough coverage on the bottom to prevent rear and side exposure.

- Check the side view to confirm that you're getting enough support on top. A tie-yourself halter, wide bottom band and sizable straps are features that help.

- Go with a low-rise waist and high-cut leg for flattering fit on the bottom.

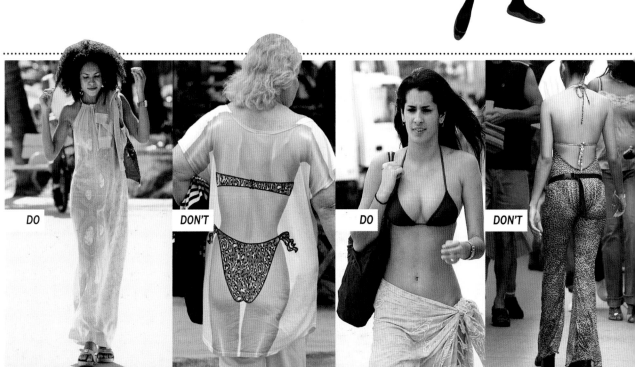

DO   DON'T   DO   DON'T

STRING BIKINI

- Choose a tie-it-yourself style—top and bottom—so you can customize fit and support.

- Look for a low-rise bottom to add curves to narrow hips.

- All cotton, in a tiny allover print, can make this style more figure-friendly.

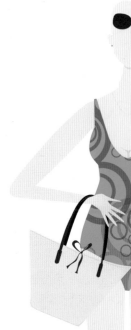

③ ONE-PIECE

- Make sure the leg opening is at the widest part of the hip; it makes your leg look longer.

- Ditch the high-neck styles you wore for swim meets; opt for a scoop- or V-neck.

- Think about a solid color with feminine details, like ruching or ruffles, to play up your curves.

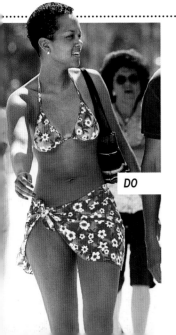

DO

Style Clinic

Cover-ups: how to be a DO

You can get away with showing a lot of skin when you're poolside, but sooner or later, you'll be headed for dry ground. Instead of settling for a T-shirt, try a sarong you can wrap any which way, a pretty tunic or even something that's already in your closet, like an oxford shirt, a denim mini or a sundress. Mesh? See-through? A faux body-double? Nope.

"I don't feel at all confident running around and eating lunch in a bikini. I'm the first person to tie a sarong around my waist."
—ELIZABETH HURLEY, ACTRESS

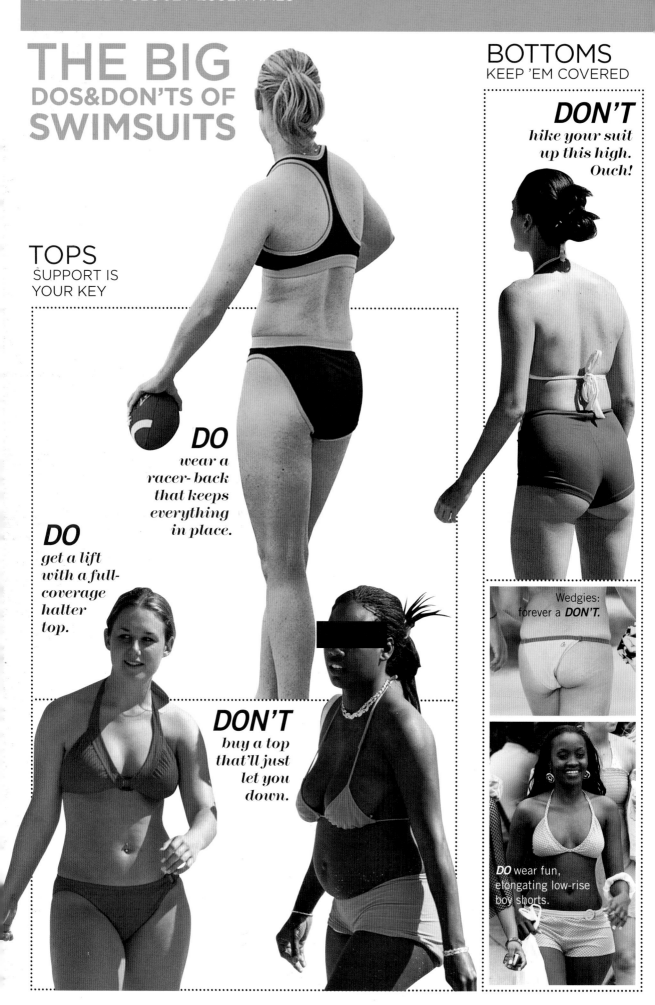

THE BIG
DOS&DON'TS OF
SWIMSUITS

TOPS
SUPPORT IS
YOUR KEY

DO
*wear a
racer-back
that keeps
everything
in place.*

DO
*get a lift
with a full-
coverage
halter
top.*

DON'T
*buy a top
that'll just
let you
down.*

BOTTOMS
KEEP 'EM COVERED

DON'T
*hike your suit
up this high.
Ouch!*

Wedgies:
forever a **DON'T.**

DO wear fun,
elongating low-rise
boy shorts.

54

PATTERNS
FOR FUN OR FLATTERY

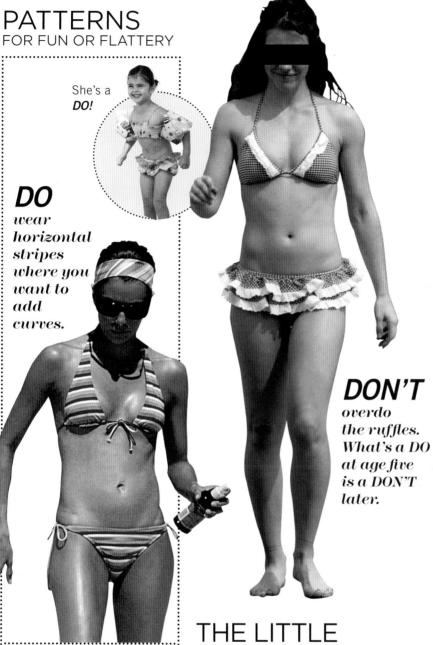

She's a **DO!**

DO
wear horizontal stripes where you want to add curves.

DON'T
overdo the ruffles. What's a DO at age five is a DON'T later.

THE LITTLE RED BIKINI
A DO THEN, A DO NOW

DO go with a classic crimson bikini like Raquel Welch's, in 1967.

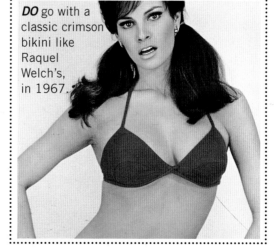

DO wear a bold allover pattern in a cut that flatters you.

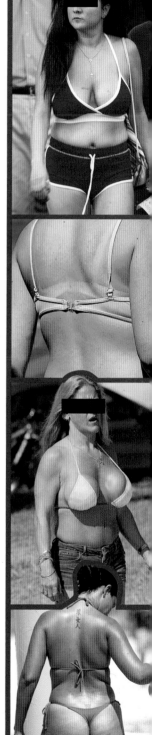

GLAMOUR FACT: BESIDES BIKINIS, EVA LONGORIA'S WEEKEND FASHION STAPLES ARE UGGS AND TRUE RELIGION JEANS.

SHOES

THREE MUST-HAVE WEEKEND SHOES

On weekends, you want total footwear comfort. Stylish comfort, of course. Three styles that deliver: cowboy boots, non-work-out sneakers and flip-flops or flat sandals.

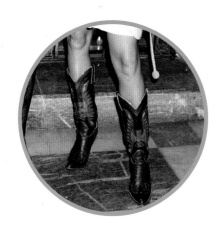

 1

COWBOY BOOTS

- Look for boots with a small heel—comfortable to run around in, but still stylish.

- Choose an almost knee-high pair that your jeans can fit over or be tucked into.

- Avoid kitschy, multicolor styles— your very safest bets are black and brown, but colorful solids work too.

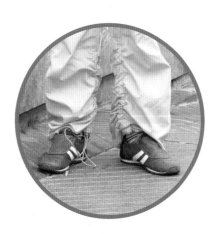

 2

SNEAKERS

- Save the clunky white ones for the gym, and wear a fun thin-soled style.

- If you're pairing 'em with skirts or capris, wear low-low socks that you can't see.

- Bright colors look cool with dark denim.

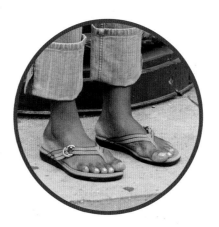

 3

SANDALS

- Try metallic or jeweled styles with dressy stuff.

- Bare sandals in bright colors can go with almost anything.

- Toss out rubber flip-flops when the soles wear down.

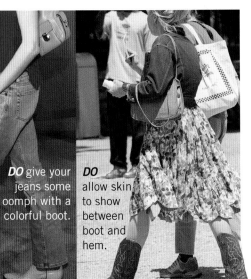

DO give your jeans some oomph with a colorful boot.

DO allow skin to show between boot and hem.

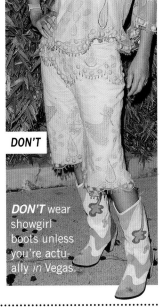

DON'T

DON'T wear showgirl boots unless you're actually *in* Vegas.

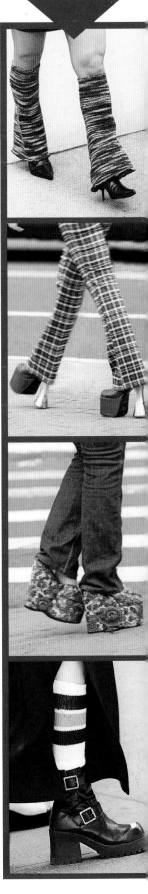

DO pair a denim skirt with funky kicks.

DO cuff your long jeans when you're wearing sneaks.

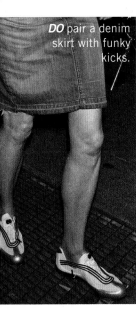

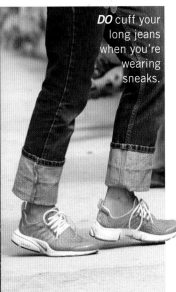

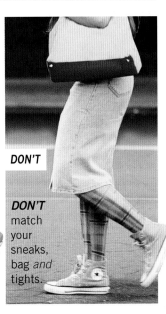

DON'T

DON'T match your sneaks, bag *and* tights.

DO wear comfy espadrilles to the beach.

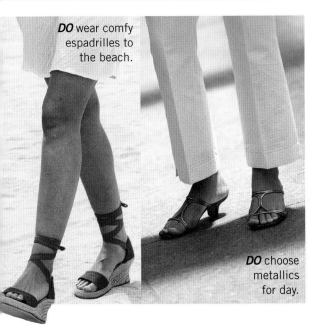

Socks with sandals? An all-time **DON'T.**

DON'T

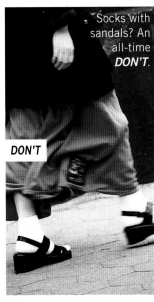

DO choose metallics for day.

HAIR

EASY, PERFECT WEEKEND HAIR

There's a time and a place for elaborate updos and 12-step hot-roller routines, but the weekend isn't it. You need styles that are lower-maintenance but still presentable: loose ponytails, beachy braids, messy buns and the like. And try scarves and head-bands—they're girlier than baseball caps, and way more flattering.

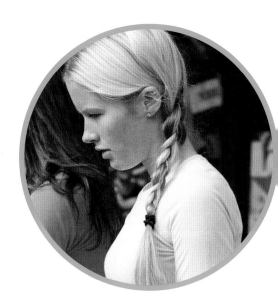

BRAID

- Wear one at a time; two is best left for the under-12 set.

- Your hair needs to be at least shoulder-length for a braid to work.

- For the most adult look, secure your 'do with elastics that match your hair.

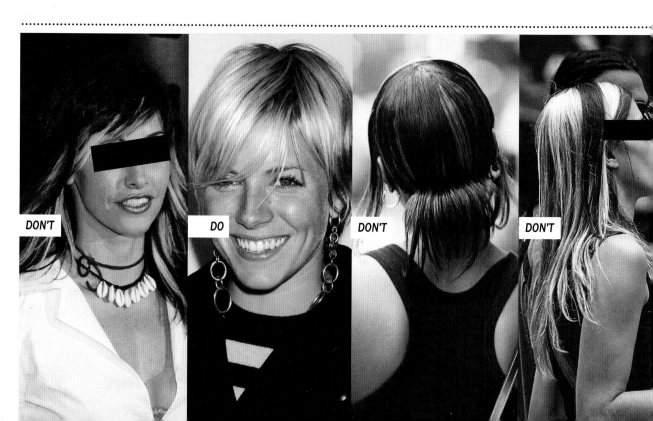

DON'T   **DO**   **DON'T**   **DON'T**

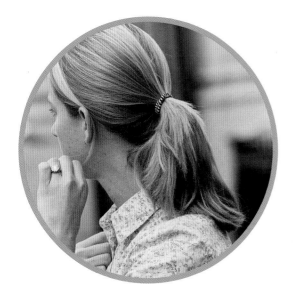

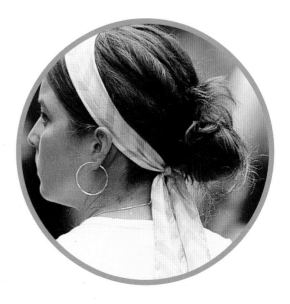

 2

PONYTAIL

- To keep the style loose, not severe, pull out a few short pieces around your face.

- Thicker, longer hair looks best in low ponytails.

- Shorter hair can go into a low, messy bun.

 3

HEADBAND

- Choose the right width. For a smaller head, a narrow band is best.

- To look very now, wear a band closer to the front of your head and keep your bangs loose.

- If you're using a scarf for this look, opt for a lightweight fabric; keep it from slipping with two bobby pins.

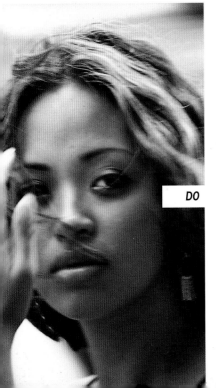

DO

Style Clinic

Highlights: how to be a DO

These days almost everyone has them—for better or worse. To keep your highlights a DO and not a DON'T, follow three simple rules: 1. Keep 'em subtle. Highlights should only differ *slightly* from your natural color. No skunk stripes. 2. Make sure they're framing your face; they look awkward in the back. 3. You don't have to obsess about your roots—those days are over—but try to touch up at least every two months.

"Gorgeous hair is the best revenge."
—IVANA TRUMP, SOCIALITE

THE BIG
DOS&DON'TS OF
HAIR

5 HAIRSTYLE TO AVOID

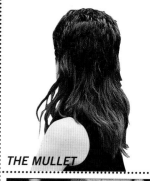

THE MULLET

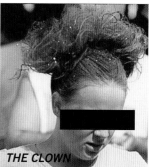

THE CLOWN

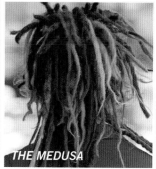

THE MEDUSA

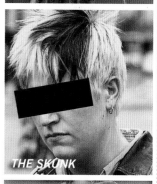

THE SKUNK

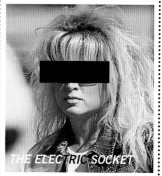

THE ELECTRIC SOCKET

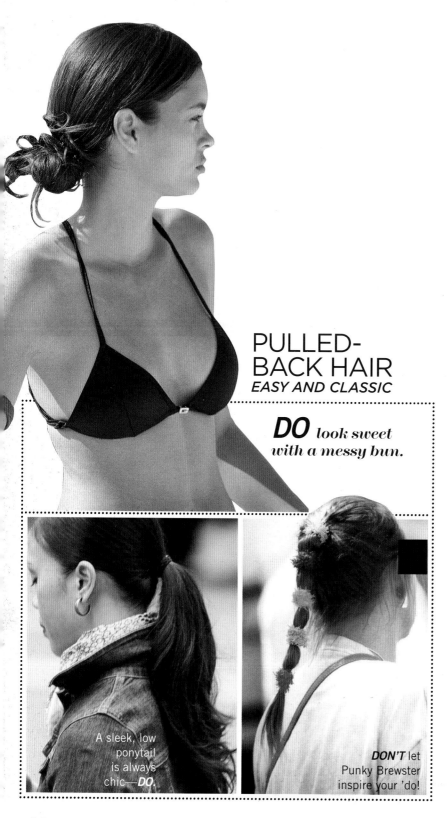

PULLED-BACK HAIR
EASY AND CLASSIC

DO *look sweet with a messy bun.*

A sleek, low ponytail is always chic—**DO**.

DON'T let Punky Brewster inspire your 'do!

GLAMOUR FACT: FAMOUS WOMEN WHO HAVE HAD MULLETS INCLUDE MELISSA ETHERIDGE, SCARLETT JOHANSSON, MILLA JOVOVICH, KAREN O OF THE YEAH YEAH YEAHS AND GWEN STEFANI.

60

ACCESSORIES:
ONE GREAT PIECE IS ALL YOU NEED

JUST DON'T!

AH, THE BAD HAIR DAY... WE'VE ALL BEEN THERE!

DO
let your scarf trail down your back.

DO
use a small clip to hold a fuss-free updo.

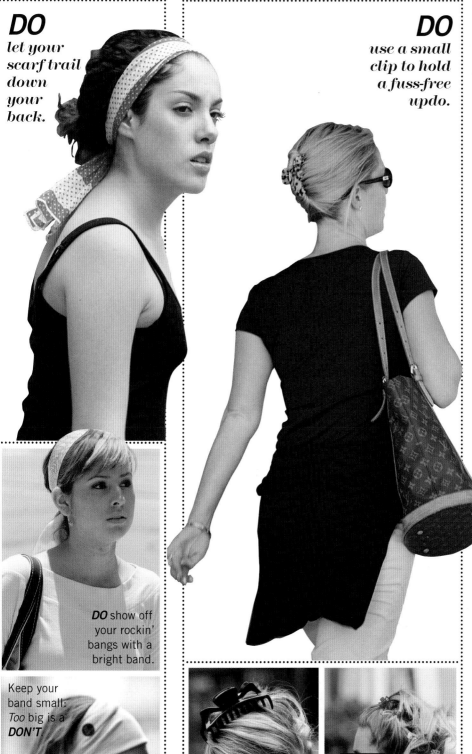

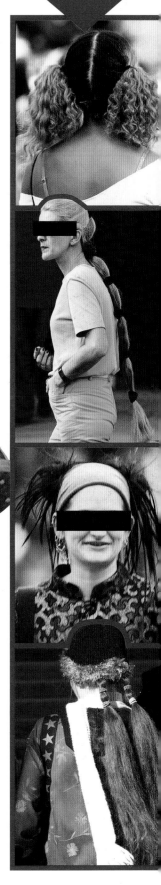

DO show off your rockin' bangs with a bright band.

Keep your band small: *Too* big is a **DON'T.**

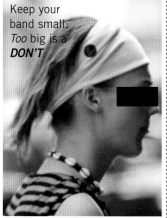

Hint: When the clip is as big as your head, it's a **DON'T.**

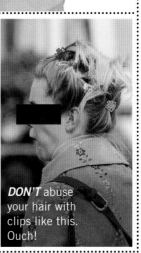

DON'T abuse your hair with clips like this. Ouch!

YOU'RE GOING AWAY FOR
THE WEEKEND

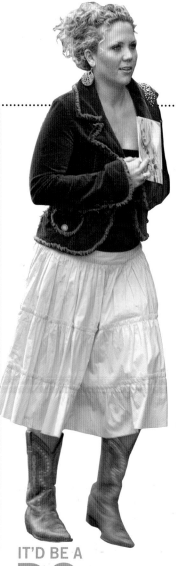

IT'D BE A
DO
BECAUSE

- A denim skirt, thick tights and tall boots are fun and urban-appropriate.
- Square, stacked heels are comfortable for walking.
- The retro, fur-collared jacket will look great with a dress at night, too.

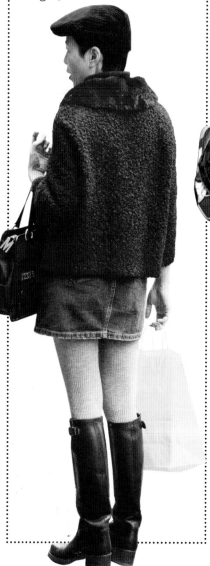

IT'D BE A
DO
BECAUSE

- Peasant skirts are perfect for travel: They're comfortable for walking and almost wrinkle-proof.
- The fitted blazer adds polish and can take the look from day to evening.
- Flat boots are more proper than sneakers but not too dressed up. (They *are* heavy to pack, though!)

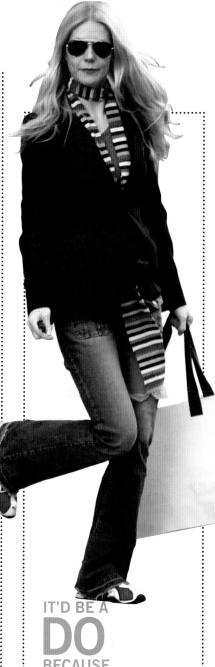

IT'D BE A
DO
BECAUSE

- Great-fitting jeans will never fail you.
- These kicks are street-smart, not gym-going.
- A tailored blazer ups the style quotient.
- A long, bright scarf gives the whole outfit personality.

OVERPACKING IS EASY; CARTING A 50-POUND BAG ONTO PLANES, trains and automobiles *isn't*. Even if your getaway activities aren't totally streamlined, your packing plans can be. The three secrets? 1. Know your destination. If you're headed for party-central Hollywood, pack dresses for the clubs. If you're spending a week at a beach resort, leave dress slacks at home. You'll live in skirts and sarongs. 2. Going sightseeing? Skip the clunky white sneakers and opt for comfy, colorful flats with a squishy sole. 3. Bring one item, like a sparkly scarf or a pair of metallic heels, that'll make whatever you pair with it look special. Oh, and one last rule: If you never wear it at home, odds are you won't wear it when you're away—so don't bother packing it.

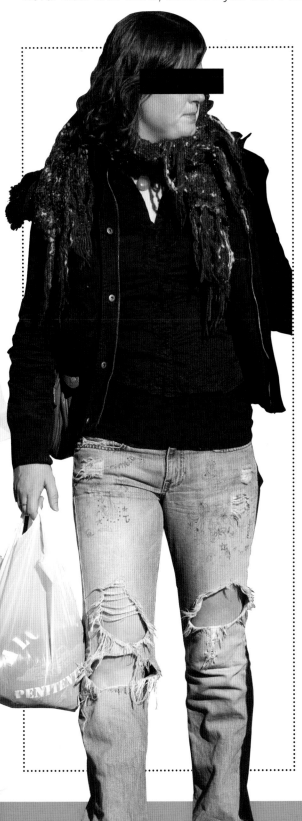

Found!

FIVE LITTLE MUST-PACK ITEMS THAT MAKE VACATIONS SPECIAL

1.
Jewelry
Take lots of baubles in your carry-on bag: Notice-me earrings and necklaces let you wear an outfit twice without feeling boring.

2.
Heels
They elevate even jeans and a cardigan to evening status.

3.
Wrap/scarf
Toss a bright color over your shoulders and you'll be glam *and* warm.

4.
Lipstick
Fire engine–red lip color makes you feel instantly done up—even without your usual 17 makeup products.

5.
Flirty lingerie
The sexy charge you get comes through no matter what you put on over it.

IT'D BE A
DON'T
BECAUSE

- This look is a no go, uh, anywhere. All those holes look like you got into a fight with the airport security dogs—and lost.
- This stringy scarf needs to be neatly tied.

YOU'RE GOING TO A BACKYARD BARBECUE

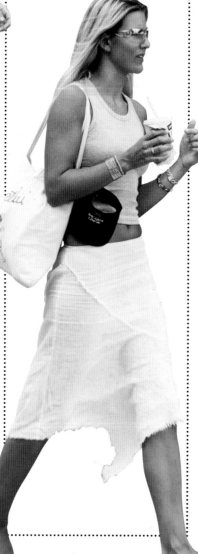

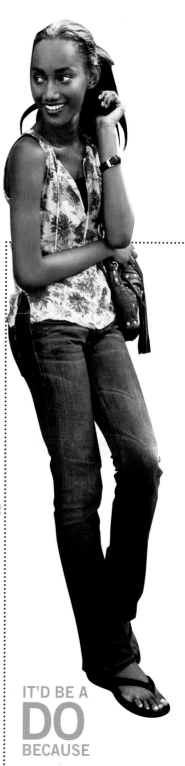

IT'D BE A
DO
BECAUSE

- A simple tank top takes the edge off a funky skirt.
- Shades are chic and protect your eyes from the sun.
- Multiple bracelets add personal style.

IT'D BE A
DO
BECAUSE

- A cotton sundress makes you feel like summer.
- The strapless neckline is just sexy enough.
- Unlike heels, flip-flops won't sink into the grass.

IT'D BE A
DO
BECAUSE

- Playing bocce ball? Sitting on the grass? Jeans'll prevent ants in your pants.
- A printed, flowy top pretties up jeans.
- Sexy pedicured toes go with any bare shoe.

GRAZING ON TASTY FOOD IN THE OPEN AIR IS AN IDEAL WAY TO SPEND A SATURDAY—so what to wear that's more stylish than your college-era cutoffs? (It *is* a party, after all.) Consider these backyard guidelines: 1. If you can't bend over to toss a football or throw your niece in the air while wearing it, skip it. 2. If it's pricey, delicate, or dry-clean only, it'll just make you nervous—skip it. You want clothes that are at least semi-resistant to mustard stains. 3. If you'd wear it on the rides at the water park, it's too casual. Yep: Skip it. What *to* wear? These DOs.

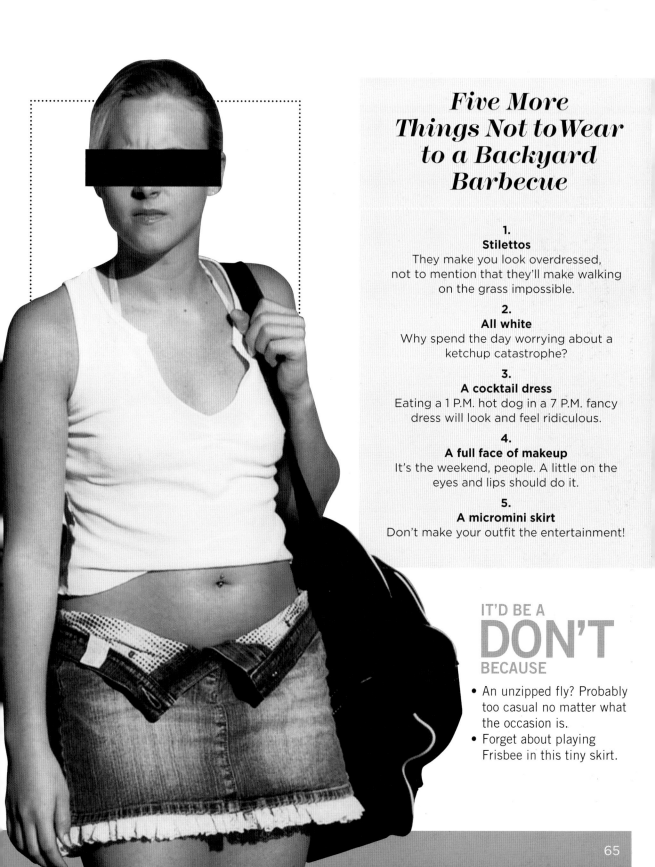

Five More Things Not to Wear to a Backyard Barbecue

1.
Stilettos
They make you look overdressed, not to mention that they'll make walking on the grass impossible.

2.
All white
Why spend the day worrying about a ketchup catastrophe?

3.
A cocktail dress
Eating a 1 P.M. hot dog in a 7 P.M. fancy dress will look and feel ridiculous.

4.
A full face of makeup
It's the weekend, people. A little on the eyes and lips should do it.

5.
A micromini skirt
Don't make your outfit the entertainment!

IT'D BE A
DON'T
BECAUSE

- An unzipped fly? Probably too casual no matter what the occasion is.
- Forget about playing Frisbee in this tiny skirt.

IS IT A DO OR A DON'T?

OVERALLS

On teddy bears and small children, overalls are adorable and functional, even stylish. On adults, though, they're a different story. Unless you're lounging around the house (or painting it), there are few appropriate occasions to wear adult versions of this "onesie." So just DON'T.

OUR VERDICT:
almost always a DON'T

DON'T
go for the tube-top-and overalls look.

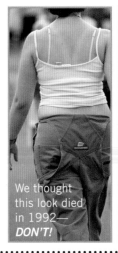

We thought this look died in 1992— **DON'T!**

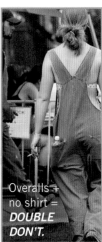

Overalls + no shirt = **DOUBLE DON'T.**

THE LONG SCARF

A long scarf is a great extra on cooler days, but make sure it isn't so long that you (or others!) are tripping over it. Extra caveat to petites: Don't let the ends hang below your knees.

OUR VERDICT:
a DO (if done right)

Winter white and just the right length: **DO**

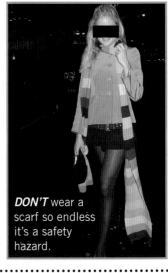

DON'T wear a scarf so endless it's a safety hazard.

MESSAGE TEES

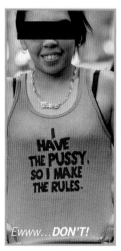

Ewww...**DON'T!**

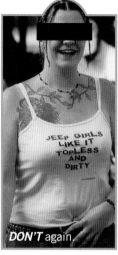

DON'T again.

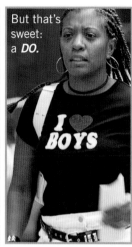

But that's sweet: a **DO**.

Being a human billboard can be sincere (*I Heart NY*), silly (*My Sister Went to Italy and All She Got Me Was This Stupid T-shirt*), political (*Support Our Troops*) or gross (these DON'Ts). But if you wouldn't say it to your niece, DON'T say it on your shirt.

OUR VERDICT:
a DON'T! (and watch what you say)

THE VELOUR SWEATSUIT

Wearing your favorite comfy sweatsuit now and then is fine—throw it on to go to the gym or run a quick errand. Just DON'T make it your weekend uniform. If you absolutely can't resist, use the pieces as separates and pair, say, the hoodie with khakis or cargo pants.

OUR VERDICT:
sometimes a DO

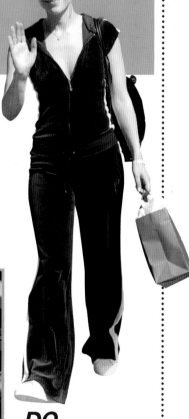

DO wear a sweatsuit to grab coffee, a paper or a long flight.

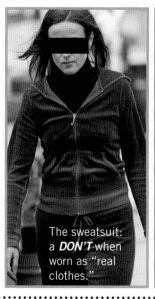

The sweatsuit: a **DON'T** when worn as "real clothes."

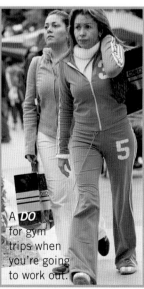

A **DO** for gym trips when you're going to work out.

"I WANT CLOTHES THAT SHOW MY FIGURE"

That's what Kacie, a chemical engineer, thought when she saw pictures of herself in the shapeless boho dress below, an old favorite from her closet. "It's lightweight, so I wear it in the summer, but clearly, it's not the most formfitting dress." To uncover her great body, she's switching to pieces that highlight her petite frame and small waist.

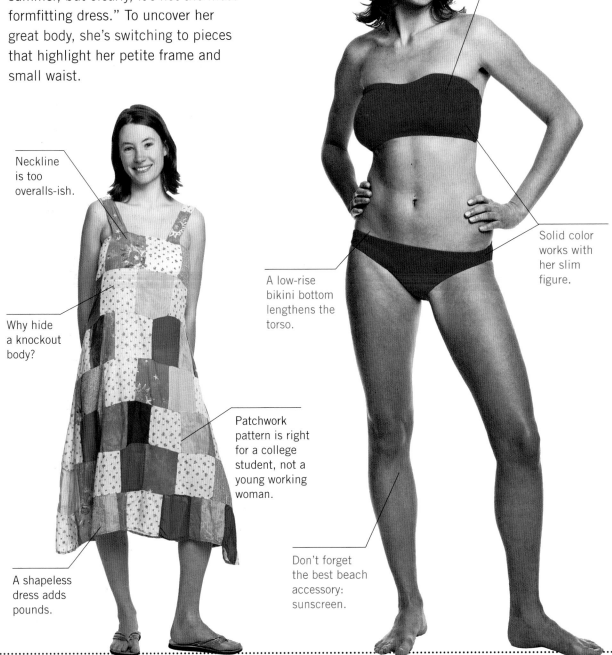

Neckline is too overalls-ish.

Why hide a knockout body?

A shapeless dress adds pounds.

Patchwork pattern is right for a college student, not a young working woman.

A bandeau with underwire inside provides support.

A low-rise bikini bottom lengthens the torso.

Solid color works with her slim figure.

Don't forget the best beach accessory: sunscreen.

BEFORE:
Kacie Fisher, 23

LOUNGING BY THE POOL

"I used to wear triangle tops, but they never gave me enough support. With a bandeau, I'm not falling out all over the place."

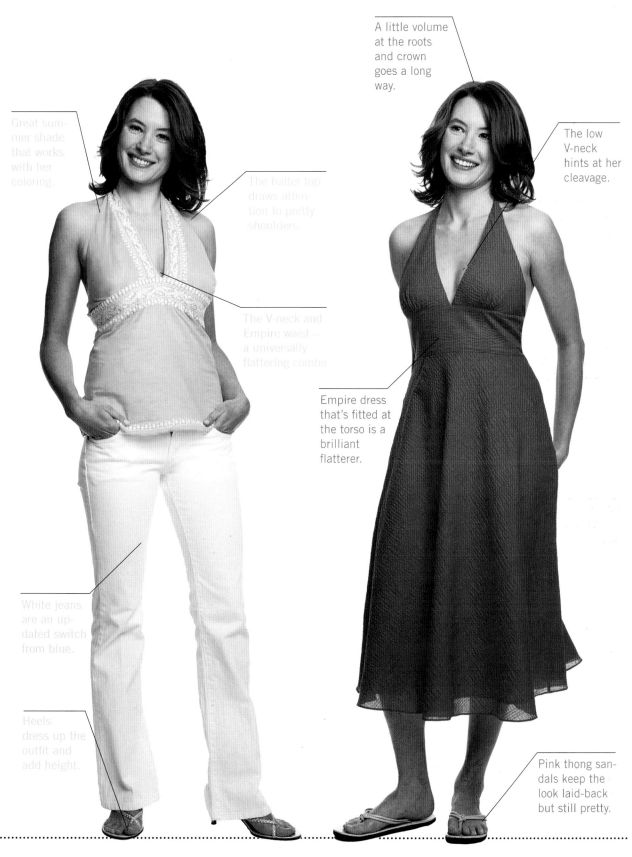

A little volume at the roots and crown goes a long way.

Great summer shade that works with her coloring.

The halter top draws attention to pretty shoulders.

The low V-neck hints at her cleavage.

The V-neck and Empire waist—a universally flattering combo.

Empire dress that's fitted at the torso is a brilliant flatterer.

White jeans are an updated switch from blue.

Heels dress up the outfit and add height.

Pink thong sandals keep the look laid-back but still pretty.

AFTER-SUNSET COCKTAILS

"This is great for having drinks on a friend's backyard deck."

DINNER ALFRESCO

"I'd wear this to a beachfront restaurant. It's not too fancy and it's much cuter than a T-shirt and shorts."

"I'M 28, NOT 18!"

"I swear I'd only wear this if I wasn't leaving the house!" says Lauren about the outfit below. Being comfortable on the weekends is paramount when this prop stylist is running around the city shopping for shoots, but so are clothes that match her age and her creative personality. Here, she's in body-conscious, go-anywhere clothes that pop with color and pizzazz.

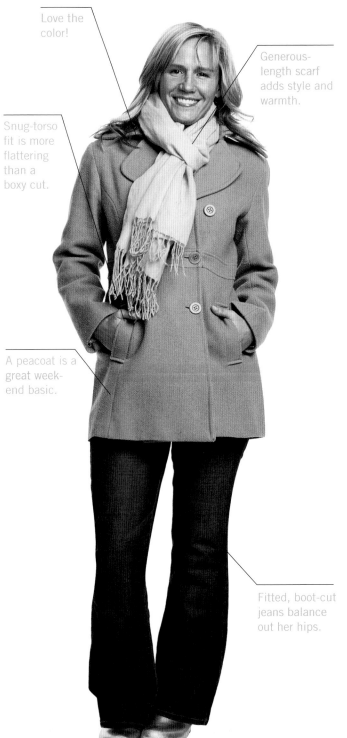

Love the color!

Generous-length scarf adds style and warmth.

Snug-torso fit is more flattering than a boxy cut.

A peacoat is a great week-end basic.

Fitted, boot-cut jeans balance out her hips.

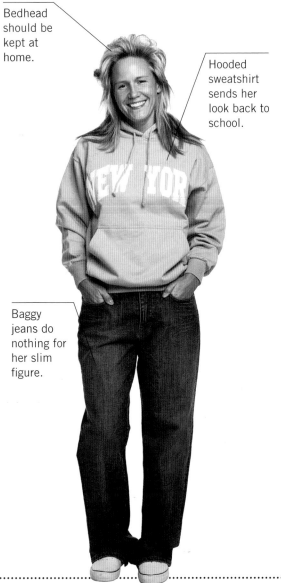

Bedhead should be kept at home.

Hooded sweatshirt sends her look back to school.

Baggy jeans do nothing for her slim figure.

BEFORE:

Lauren Shields, 28

SATURDAY SHOPPING

"Warm enough for going outside; fun enough for flea-market shopping!"

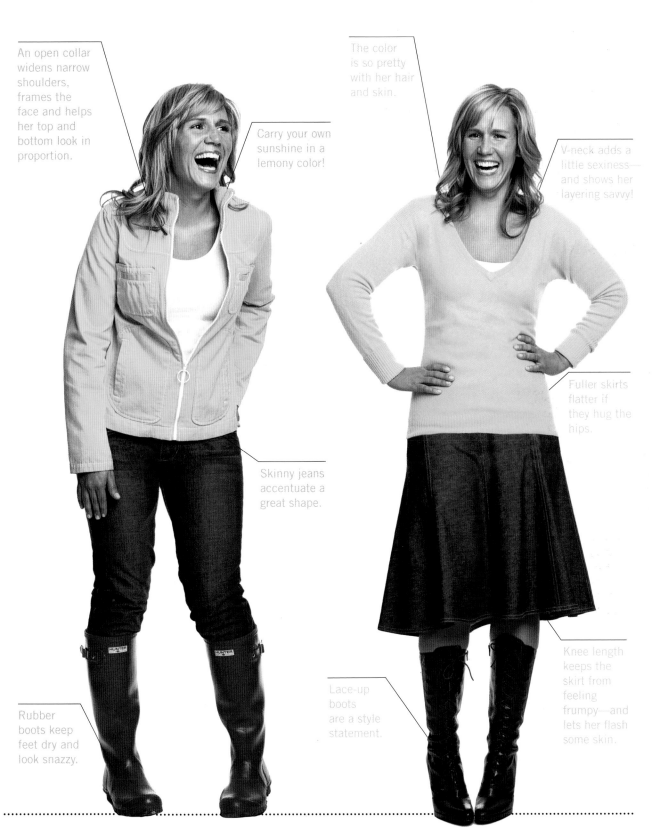

An open collar widens narrow shoulders, frames the face and helps her top and bottom look in proportion.

Carry your own sunshine in a lemony color!

The color is so pretty with her hair and skin.

V-neck adds a little sexiness—and shows her layering savvy!

Skinny jeans accentuate a great shape.

Fuller skirts flatter if they hug the hips.

Rubber boots keep feet dry and look snazzy.

Lace-up boots are a style statement.

Knee length keeps the skirt from feeling frumpy—and lets her flash some skin.

RUNNING ERRANDS

"This outfit proves you can even look cute on a rainy day!"

FRIEND'S HOUSE PARTY

"It's dressy, but still casual; good for seeing friends."

"SHOW OFF MY CURVES, PLEASE"

Buried beneath all the too-big clothes in this student's closet, we found a sexy body ready to make its debut. Says Jordan of her baggy outfit, below, "I thought the wide-legged pants would minimize my thighs and the sweater would cover up my large bust." Here, her new clothes help accentuate her positives, not cover them up.

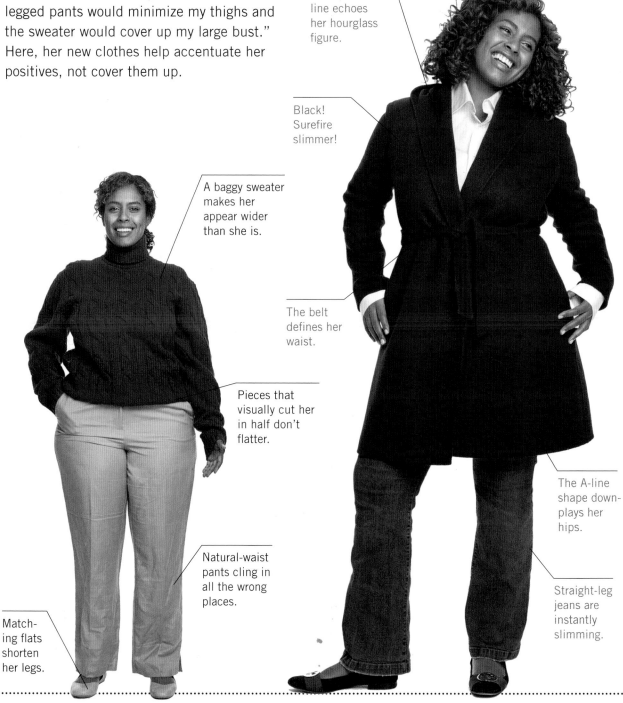

A deep neck-line echoes her hourglass figure.

Black! Surefire slimmer!

A baggy sweater makes her appear wider than she is.

The belt defines her waist.

Pieces that visually cut her in half don't flatter.

The A-line shape down-plays her hips.

Natural-waist pants cling in all the wrong places.

Straight-leg jeans are instantly slimming.

Match-ing flats shorten her legs.

BEFORE:
Jordan Tesfay, 26

LUNCH WITH THE GIRLS

"I don't try to hide my butt, but I'm OK with not maximizing it!"

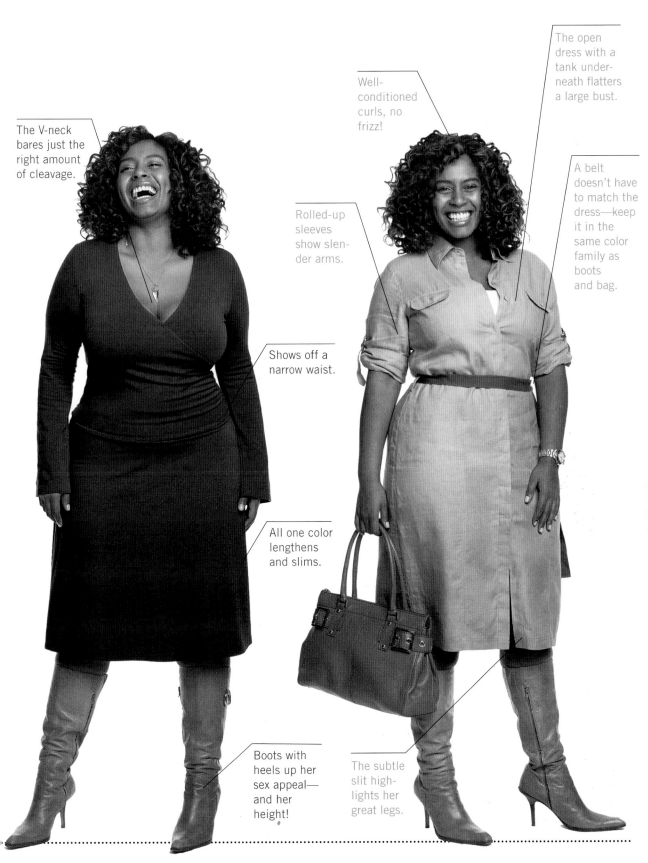

The V-neck bares just the right amount of cleavage.

Well-conditioned curls, no frizz!

The open dress with a tank underneath flatters a large bust.

Rolled-up sleeves show slender arms.

A belt doesn't have to match the dress—keep it in the same color family as boots and bag.

Shows off a narrow waist.

All one color lengthens and slims.

Boots with heels up her sex appeal—and her height!

The subtle slit highlights her great legs.

DINNER À DEUX

"Great for a dinner date. The dress accents my curves and small waist!"

OFF TO WORK

"This is so comfortable and it totally works with my body shape."

HALL
OF
shame

EXTREME SWIMSUIT DON'TS
YIKES! LOOK OUT BELOW (AND ABOVE)!

DON'T pick a top that lets this happen.

DON'T let your suit stay this wedged.

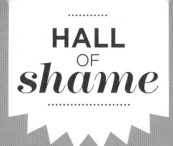

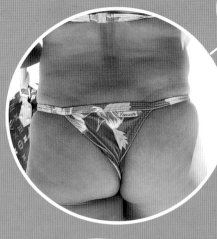

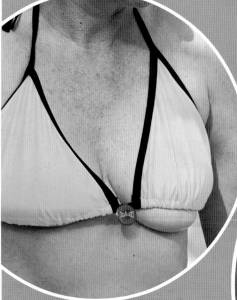

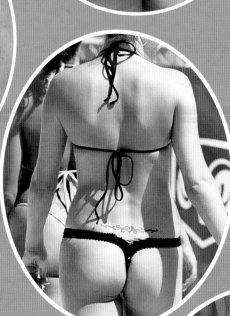

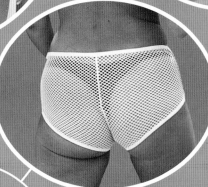

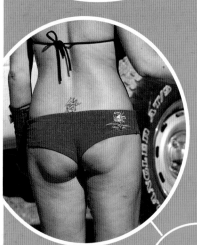

Even if your bikini is in the wash, ***DON'T*** wear your thong as a swimsuit.

DON'T forget the bottom half of your bum!

DON'T do mesh—it just never works.

DON'T pick a top that was a vine in its previous life.

DON'T show the public your private piercings.

DON'T become this intimate with a leather seat, or any seat.

DON'T wear a bikini top that highlights your tan line.

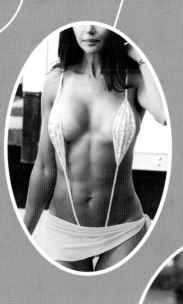

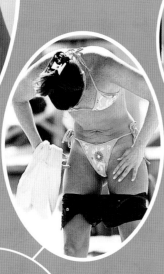

Only a slice of your breasts? That's a **DON'T**.

DON'T wait until you hit the beach to check your bikini line.

If your pants are this low, **DON'T** even bother wearing 'em.

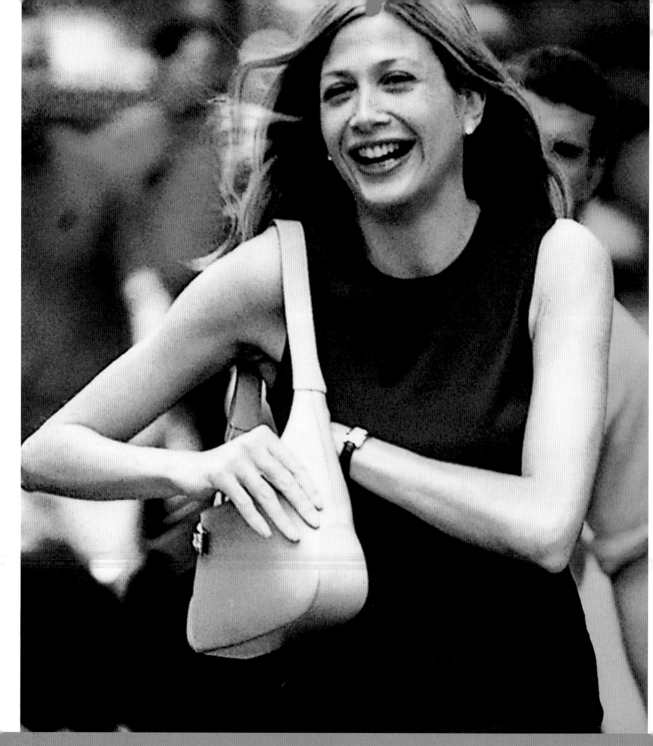

YOUR

DO

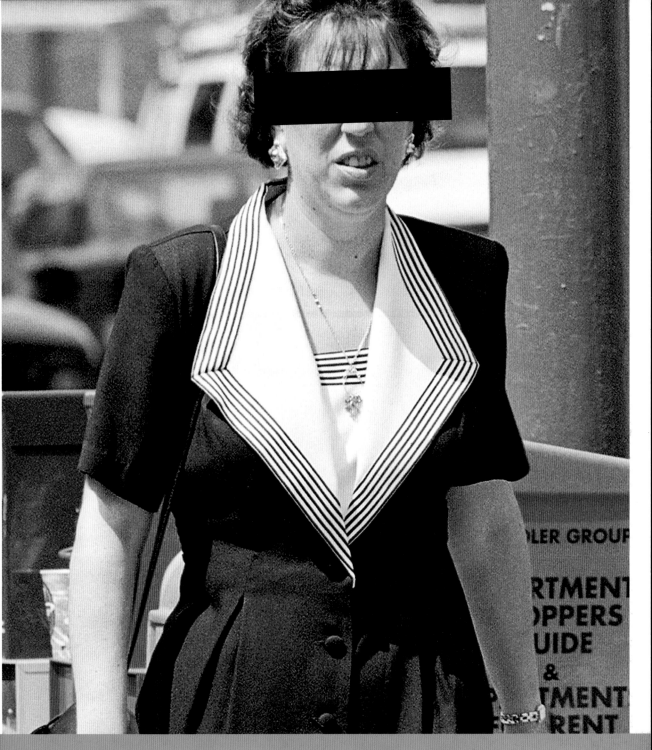

WORK LIFE

WHAT SUCCEEDS—AND WHAT DOESN'T—
IN YOUR WORLD

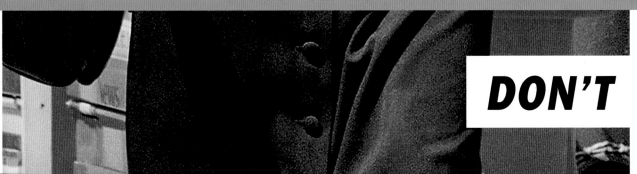

DON'T

THE RULES
for work

1

FOLLOW YOUR COMPANY'S UNOFFICIAL DRESS CODE...

You want to look like you belong, so take fashion cues from your most respected coworkers.

2

...BUT REMEMBER, IT'S OK TO SHOW A LITTLE PERSONALITY.

A winning work-style strategy: Keep the clothes simple and let your accessories shine. Bring on the chic flats, colorful heels and quirky jewelry.

3

DON'T FEEL THAT YOU NEED TO SHOW UP IN A DIFFERENT OUTFIT EVERY SINGLE DAY.

Nobody will notice that you wore the same skirt-and-blouse combo last Monday—unless it was a serious DON'T. An easy way to freshen a look? Add something new, like a colorful scarf or a wide belt.

4

WHEN IN DOUBT, GO MORE CONSERVATIVE.

Before you leave for work, look in the mirror. If you're wary of that psychedelic blouse, save it for Saturday night. Make sure to keep these perennial 9-to-5 DOs handy: a twinset, a pencil skirt and a great-fitting pair of black pants.

WEAR JEANS SPARINGLY.

*Unless you work in a super-casual environment,
limit yourself to once a week. Pick a dark pair and
wear them with a fitted jacket and dressy shoes.*

REMEMBER: A BLACK CARDIGAN
IS YOUR BFF (BEST FASHION FRIEND).

*It will protect you against subarctic AC and add a layer
of respectability to sleeveless or sheer tops.*

IF YOU CAN FOLLOW ONLY ONE RULE, THIS IS IT!

DRESS FOR THE JOB YOU WANT,
NOT THE ONE YOU HAVE.

*Pay attention to what your boss wears and echo it.
And once you've mastered that look, set your sights higher:
What's your boss's boss—or the most senior woman
in your company—got on?*

HUNT DOWN A FABULOUS BAG;
IT WILL INSTANTLY PUNCH UP
ANY OUTFIT.

Same goes for shoes—a high-quality splurge is so worth it.

PREPARE YOURSELF
FOR FASHION EMERGENCIES.

*You never know when an important meeting will pop up.
Keep good earrings, a nice necklace, a pair of heels
and a basic black or white top (in case of spilled-
coffee moments) at your desk.*

DON'T FORGET YOUR
MOST IMPORTANT ACCESSORY
(HINT: IT'S ON YOUR HEAD).

*Just like jewelry, your hair can dress up or dress down your
outfit, so make it look as good as the rest of you.*

TOPS

THREE WORK TOPS EVERY WOMAN SHOULD OWN

These basic shapes work with everything from skirts to jeans to suits. So if you're building an office wardrobe, start here. The one rule to follow: Avoid baggy shapes—they read sloppy.

TURTLENECK

- Find one made of a cotton/ Lycra blend or wool—anything made entirely of slinky, stretchy fabrics will reveal your body's every wrinkle.

- Look for one that's long and thin enough to tuck in, and throw on a jacket and belt to go instantly conservative.

- Pair it with all kinds of bottoms, from wide-leg trousers to miniskirts and tights.

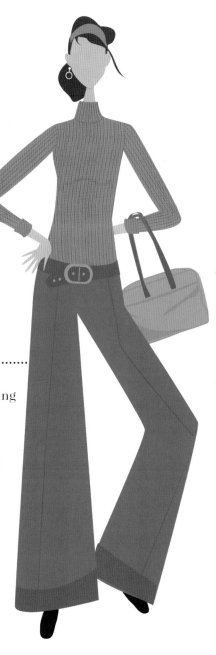

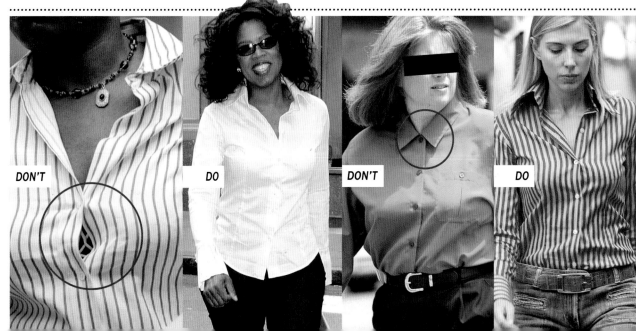

DON'T

DO

DON'T

DO

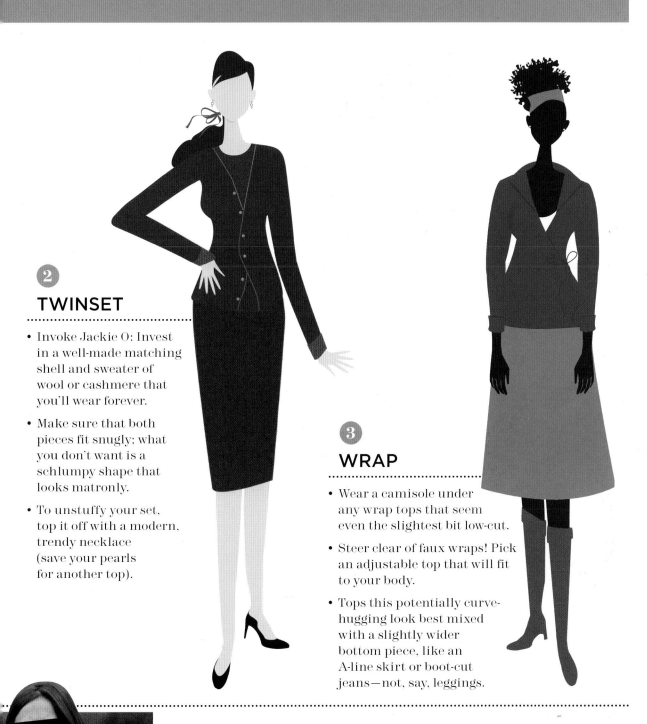

② TWINSET

- Invoke Jackie O: Invest in a well-made matching shell and sweater of wool or cashmere that you'll wear forever.

- Make sure that both pieces fit snugly; what you don't want is a schlumpy shape that looks matronly.

- To unstuffy your set, top it off with a modern, trendy necklace (save your pearls for another top).

③ WRAP

- Wear a camisole under any wrap tops that seem even the slightest bit low-cut.

- Steer clear of faux wraps! Pick an adjustable top that will fit to your body.

- Tops this potentially curve-hugging look best mixed with a slightly wider bottom piece, like an A-line skirt or boot-cut jeans—not, say, leggings.

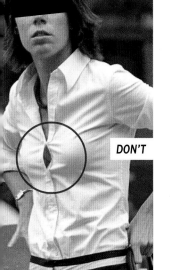

DON'T

Style Clinic

Button-down shirts: how to keep 'em closed

Everyone needs a close-fitting button-down shirt, but how can you keep them from gaping open at your bust? Bottom line: Just don't buy too tight. Your safest bet? Choose a shirt in a size that safely closes around your chest, and have it taken in everywhere else.

P.S. Don't button it all the way to the top!

"Your outward image is critical in reminding people that you have control." —CONDOLEEZZA RICE, SECRETARY OF STATE

THE BIG
DOS&DON'TS OF
TOPS

SHEER
TRICKY BUT DOABLE

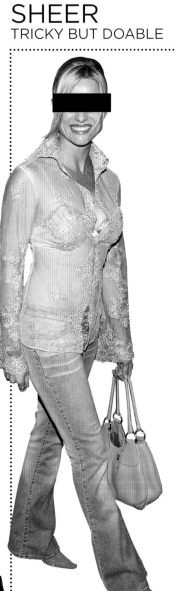

AVOID
TOO MUCH SKIN!

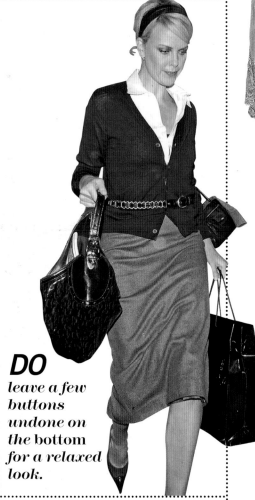

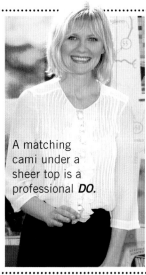

DO
leave a few buttons undone on the bottom for a relaxed look.

DON'T
show your bra— no matter how pretty it may be.

DO
top a filmy blouse with a jacket.

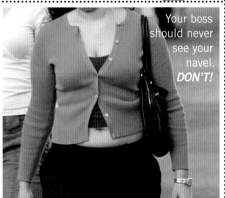

Your boss should never see your navel. **DON'T!**

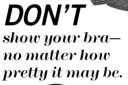

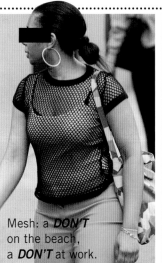

Mesh: a **DON'T** on the beach, a **DON'T** at work.

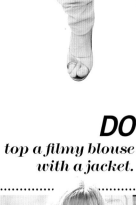

A matching cami under a sheer top is a professional **DO.**

GLAMOUR FACT: KIRSTEN DUNST (ABOVE RIGHT) WORE A JOHN GALLIANO GOWN TO HER PROM, WHICH SHE BORROWED FROM SOFIA COPPOLA. CAN-YOU-STAND-IT P.S.: HER DATE WAS JOSH HARTNETT.

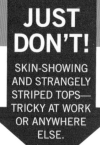

JUST DON'T!

SKIN-SHOWING AND STRANGELY STRIPED TOPS— TRICKY AT WORK OR ANYWHERE ELSE.

RED
THE POWER COLOR

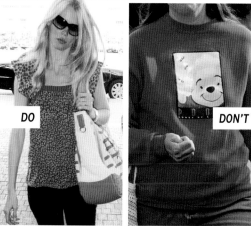

DO

DON'T

FITTED TURTLENECK
A CLASSIC DO

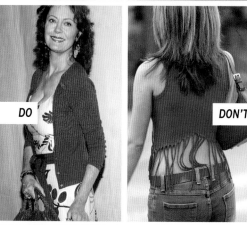

DO

DON'T

DO
dress yours up with sleek pants and a smile.

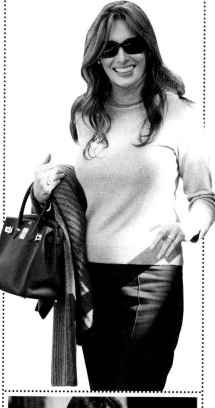

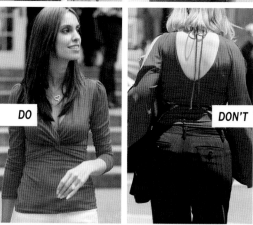

DO

DON'T

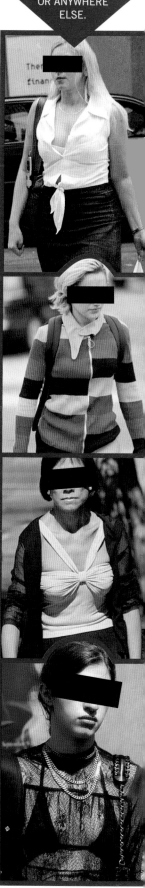

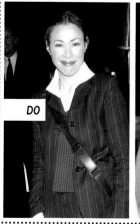

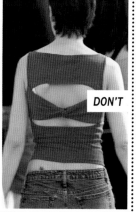

DO

DON'T

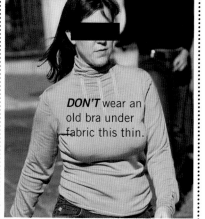

DON'T wear an old bra under fabric this thin.

SKIRTS

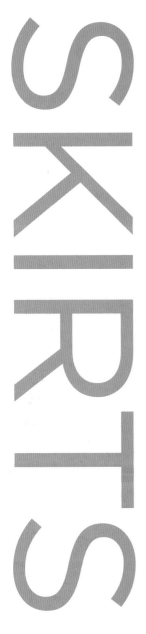

THREE SMART SKIRT SHAPES FOR WORK

When it comes to work skirts, too short is an automatic DON'T. Unsure if yours is skimpy? It should be no more than three inches above your kneecaps, max—and in conservative fields like law, banking and medicine, even longer.

1

SHORT

- For work, choose a style with a slight A-line, not skintight, shape.

- Make sure that you pair it with a full-coverage top; turtlenecks work well. No tanks!

- The shorter the mini, the more covered your legs should be: Opaque tights with low-heeled boots are safest—switch to a higher style for going out after work.

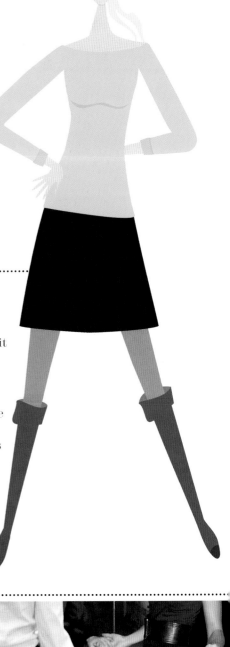

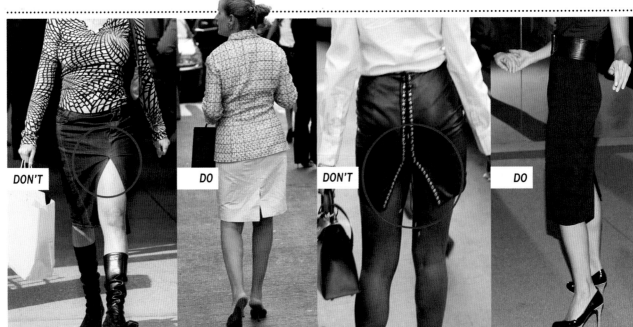

DON'T   DO   DON'T   DO

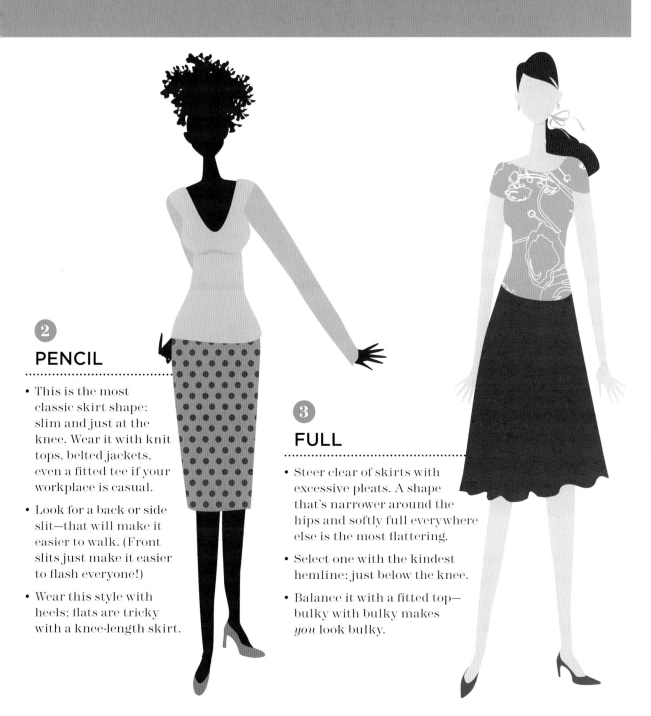

② PENCIL

- This is the most classic skirt shape: slim and just at the knee. Wear it with knit tops, belted jackets, even a fitted tee if your workplace is casual.

- Look for a back or side slit—that will make it easier to walk. (Front slits just make it easier to flash everyone!)

- Wear this style with heels; flats are tricky with a knee-length skirt.

③ FULL

- Steer clear of skirts with excessive pleats. A shape that's narrower around the hips and softly full everywhere else is the most flattering.

- Select one with the kindest hemline: just below the knee.

- Balance it with a fitted top— bulky with bulky makes *you* look bulky.

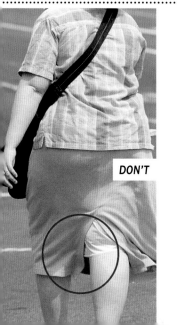

DON'T

Style Clinic

Slits: Are they a DO or a DON'T?

A well-placed slit makes walking in a fitted skirt easier—but who *hasn't* had an accidental thigh-high reveal? Ward off any potential embarrassment in the dressing room. When you're standing, the slit should lie flat, not gape open. And check where it hits when you sit and cross your legs—the real moment of truth.

"Slit skirts have a classic sexiness . . . with the unexpected flash of leg. You think you're seeing something that you're not supposed to." —**CYNTHIA ROWLEY, DESIGNER**

DRESSES

THREE CLASSIC WORK DRESSES

They couldn't be easier to wear—and they transition seamlessly from day to evening. Keep them basic at the office, and dress 'em up at night. All it takes is some heels and a bauble or two.

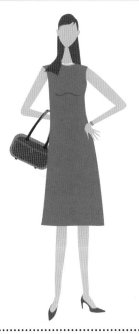

1 SHIFT DRESS

- You want to find one that is fitted but not boxy. (Darts help!)

- Also, make sure that the armholes are cut high enough to hide your bra.

- Top it off with a cardigan or short jacket (but not a long blazer, which will make you look short).

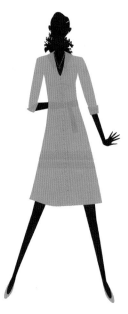

2 SHIRT DRESS

- Choose the best-fitting shape: a slim-cut top with a slightly A-line skirt.

- For a more feminine look, define your middle with a belt.

- Try strappy sandals or pumps; flats can look dowdy with this dress style.

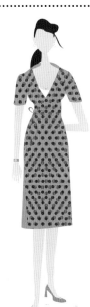

3 WRAP DRESS

- Go for fluid knits that will drape over curves, not cling to them.

- Let a cami hide your cleavage— wraps like to come untied.

- Finish with heels for a professional look; wraps can look too casual otherwise.

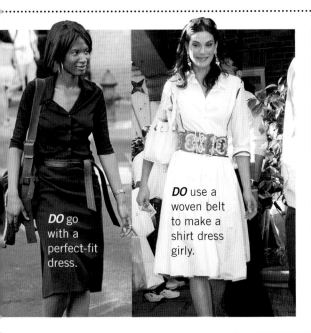

The fitted shift: a **DO**.

DO invest in a black sheath.

DON'T

DON'T wear a too-short shift with sneakers.

JUST DON'T!

DRESSES THAT ARE TOO MODEST, OR NOT MODEST ENOUGH, ARE TOUGH TO WEAR.

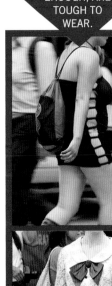

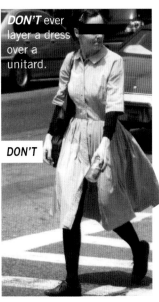

DO go with a perfect-fit dress.

DO use a woven belt to make a shirt dress girly.

DON'T ever layer a dress over a unitard.

DON'T

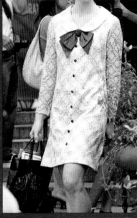

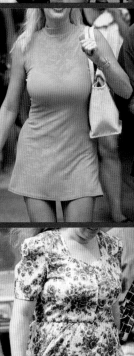

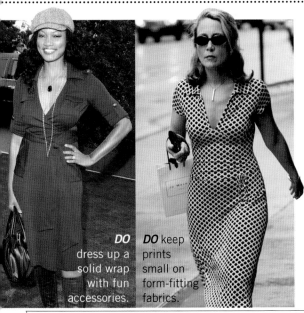

DO dress up a solid wrap with fun accessories.

DO keep prints small on form-fitting fabrics.

DON'T

Wearing Saran Wrap: a **DON'T**.

GLAMOUR FACT: SINCE DESIGNER DIANE VON FURSTENBERG INVENTED THE WRAP DRESS IN 1974, APPROXIMATELY 6 MILLION HAVE BEEN SOLD.

THE BIG
DOS&DON'TS OF
SKIRTS &
DRESSES

USE
PATTERNS
SPARINGLY

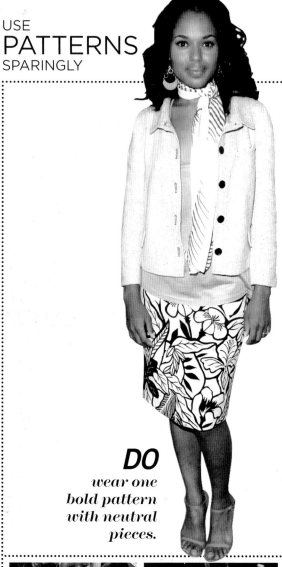

DO
wear one bold pattern with neutral pieces.

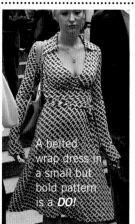

A belted wrap dress in a small but bold pattern is a *DO!*

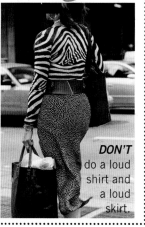

DON'T do a loud shirt and a loud skirt.

PENCIL SKIRTS?
ALSO CLASSY

DO
take a cue from Marilyn, below: This look—from 1952—is just as right on Renée today!

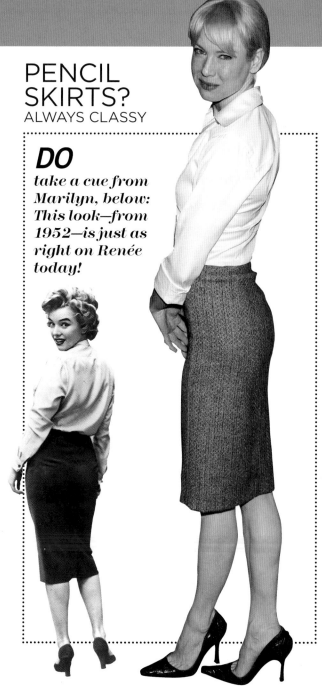

WITH MINISKIRTS,
LESS ISN'T MORE

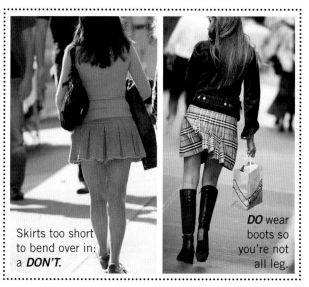

Skirts too short to bend over in: a ***DON'T.***

DO wear boots so you're not all leg.

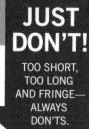

JUST DON'T!

TOO SHORT,
TOO LONG
AND FRINGE—
ALWAYS
DON'TS.

FIND
THE BEST SHAPE
FOR YOUR BODY

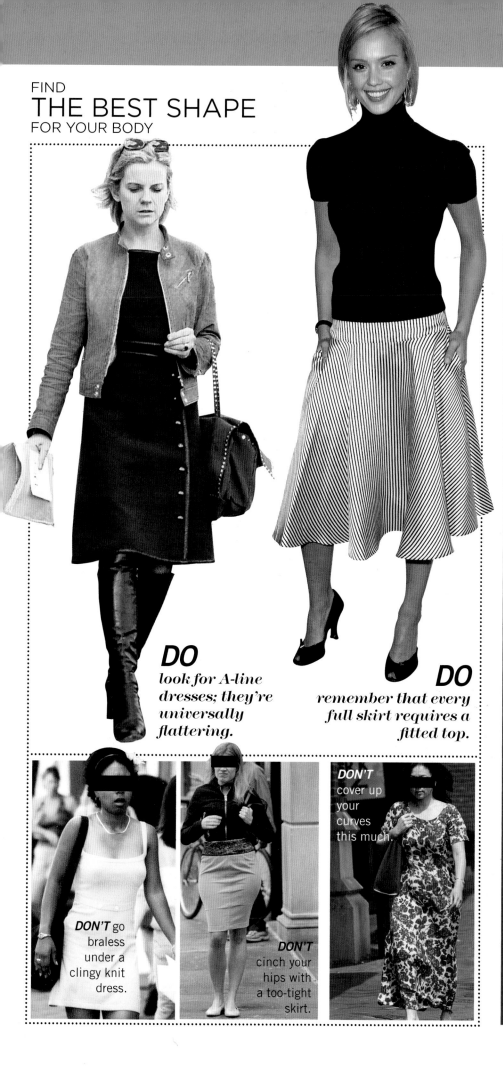

DO
*look for A-line
dresses; they're
universally
flattering.*

DO
*remember that every
full skirt requires a
fitted top.*

DON'T go
braless
under a
clingy knit
dress.

DON'T
cinch your
hips with
a too-tight
skirt.

DON'T
cover up
your
curves
this much.

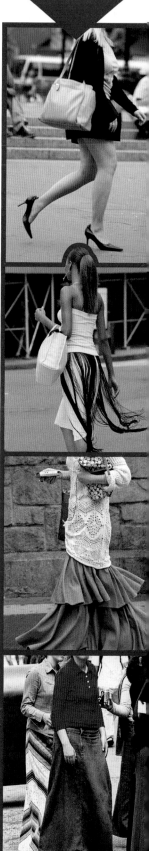

89

DENIM

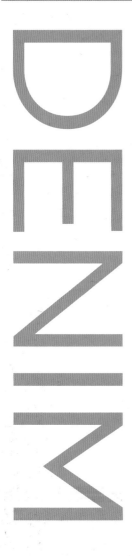

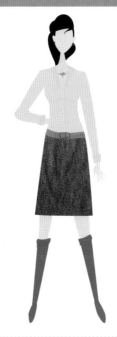

① JEANS SKIRT

- Choose a skirt that hits at the knee or right above it.

- To keep the look from being too casual, wear a button-down blouse or a jacket and camisole.

- Limit any embroidery or embellishment to just small touches, and stay away from cargo side pockets. They're too casual.

② JEANS WITH A BLAZER

- Go for midrise, straight-leg jeans in a deep, uniform color.

- Make them look trousery by wearing a shapely jacket on top.

- Finish with heels to elongate your legs.

THREE WAYS TO WEAR DENIM TO WORK

Except for weddings and funerals, denim can go anywhere these days—and that includes most workplaces. But not every piece you own should make it through the door. As a general rule, go dark and tailored. Then choose styles that mimic tried-and-true professional shapes: trouserlike jeans with straight- or boot-cut legs, fitted blazerish denim jackets and A-line or straight skirts.

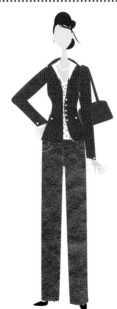

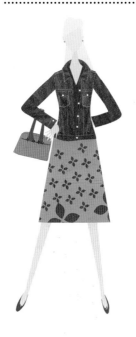

③ JEANS JACKET

- Steer clear of big, man-style cuts. Opt instead for a sleek blazer or a cropped, fitted style.

- Look feminine by wearing with skirts or dresses and heels.

- Save your faded jackets for weekends.

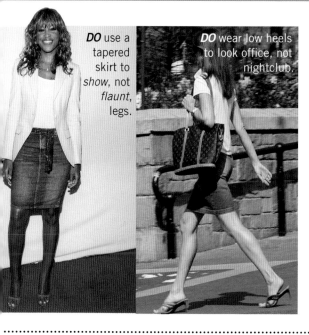

DO use a tapered skirt to *show*, not *flaunt*, legs.

DO wear low heels to look office, not nightclub.

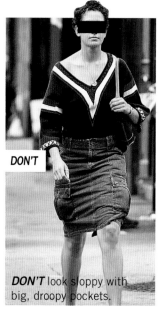

DON'T

DON'T look sloppy with big, droopy pockets.

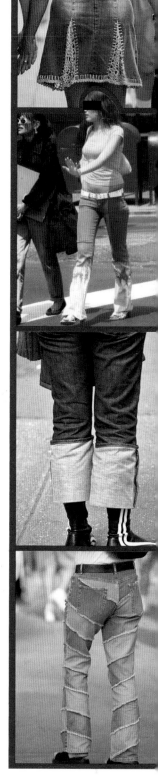

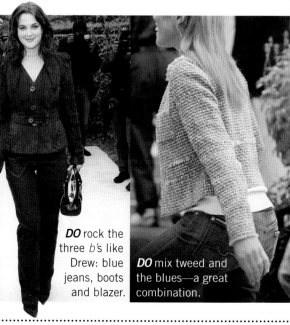

DO rock the three *b*'s like Drew: blue jeans, boots and blazer.

DO mix tweed and the blues—a great combination.

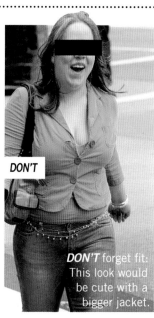

DON'T

DON'T forget fit: This look would be cute with a bigger jacket.

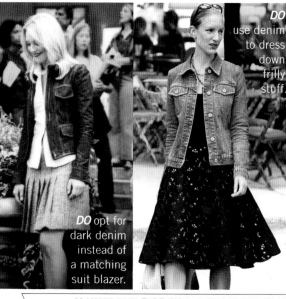

DO opt for dark denim instead of a matching suit blazer.

DO use denim to dress down frilly stuff.

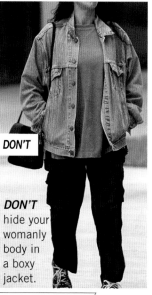

DON'T

DON'T hide your womanly body in a boxy jacket.

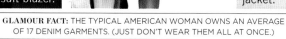

GLAMOUR FACT: THE TYPICAL AMERICAN WOMAN OWNS AN AVERAGE OF 17 DENIM GARMENTS. (JUST DON'T WEAR THEM ALL AT ONCE.)

PANTS

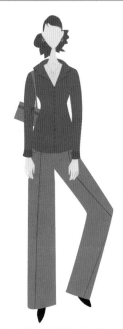

① TROUSER PANTS

- Look for flat-front styles with a medium to low rise; big pleats are bulky and unflattering.

- If you're petite, avoid wider, cuffed pants, which make legs look shorter.

- Wearing heels? Have your pants hemmed so they fall about a half inch from the ground.

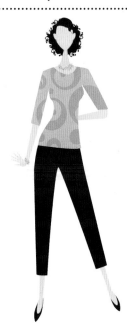

② CROPPED PANTS

- Follow this simple rule: Short pants at work should always be sleek and tailored.

- The only flattering lengths for capris: a few inches above the ankle or right below the knee.

- Finish with stacked or wedge heels to elongate legs.

THE ESSENTIAL OFFICE PANTS

Remember the day when women couldn't wear pants to work? Nope, neither can we—and neither, we bet, can your boss. These days, a great-fitting pair is a professional lifesaver. Of the three basic cuts, trouser styles are the most universally flattering. DO add heels to make your silhouette more shapely.

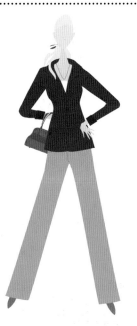

③ SLIM PANTS

- Make sure the rise is high enough to cover your butt and your belly.

- If you're pear-shaped, avoid side-zip pants; the expanse of fabric in front makes you look wider.

- Sew pockets closed for a super-sleek look.

JUST DON'T!

PANTS SO CRAZY YOU COULDN'T EVEN WEAR THEM ON CASUAL FRIDAYS.

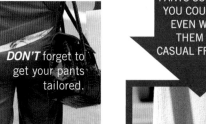

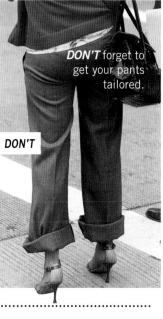

DO dress up trousers with a skinny belt and heels.

DO wear pants with cool details like flap pockets.

DON'T forget to get your pants tailored.

DON'T

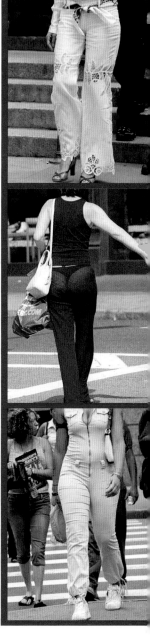

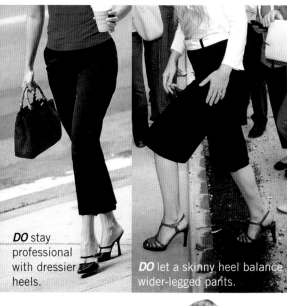

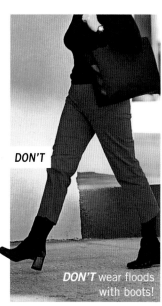

DO stay professional with dressier heels.

DO let a skinny heel balance wider-legged pants.

DON'T

DON'T wear floods with boots!

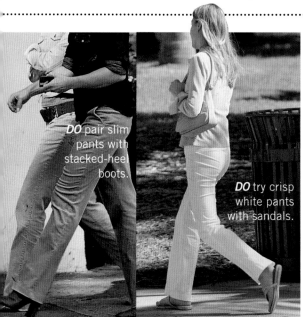

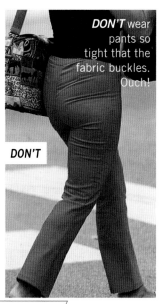

DO pair slim pants with stacked-heel boots.

DO try crisp white pants with sandals.

DON'T wear pants so tight that the fabric buckles. Ouch!

DON'T

GLAMOUR FACT: IN 1990, U.S. REP. SUSAN MOLINARI (R–N.Y.) WAS THE FIRST WOMAN TO WEAR PANTS ON THE FLOOR OF THE HOUSE.

93

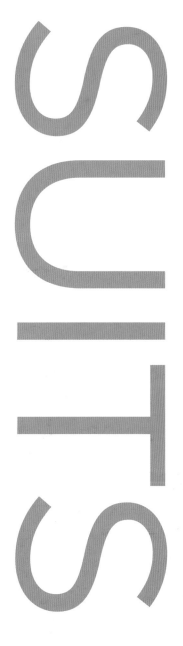

THREE CHIC SUIT STYLES

Today's suits are not the football-shoulder-padded power combos of the eighties—they're fitted, flattering and feminine. Wondering about collars? A basic lapel—as shown here, neither too wide nor too skinny—is most timeless.

PANTSUIT

- The most all-around flattering jacket length is at the hipbone or *just* below. Anything longer can look schlumpy (unless you're blessed with super-long legs).

- For the most timeless, classic style, stick with a single-breasted, narrow-lapel jacket and sleek, not overly full pants.

- And for underneath? Try a shell, unflimsy camisole or silky blouse.

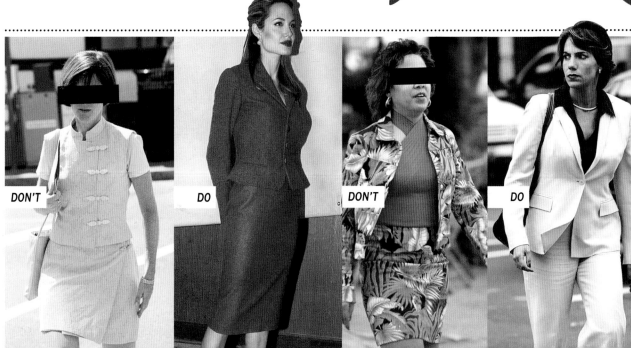

DON'T   DO   DON'T   DO

② COAT OVER DRESS

- Start with a slim shift dress that hits just at or below the knee.

- Make sure that the topper is a fitted shape and slightly shorter than the dress (so you don't look too mumsy).

- Finish with medium-height heels; flats can be dowdy.

③ SKIRT SUIT

- Beware the shapeless jacket! What you want is something that nips in a bit at the waist to show your shape.

- Choose a suit with a skirt that hits at the knee—not far above or below.

- Finish with heels to keep the proportions balanced.

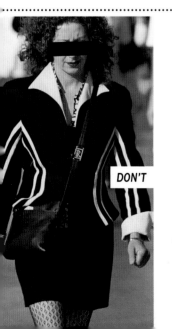

DON'T

Style Clinic

Your #1 rule for suits: Keep 'em classic

Save the hot colors, crazy fabrics, loud prints and creative details for your tops and accessories. Suits can be the priciest part of your work wardrobe, so go for neutral colors and perfect fits that you'll wear for years.

"What you wear to the office should say you're there for business, not for sex."
— ANN RICHARDS, FORMER GOVERNOR OF TEXAS

THE BIG
DOS&DON'TS OF
SUITS

THE MANSUIT
LEAVE TIES TO THE GUYS

BOLD COLOR
A BRIGHT IDEA!

PATTERNS
NICE WHEN THEY'R SUBTLE

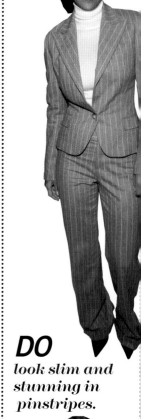

DO
look slim and stunning in pinstripes.

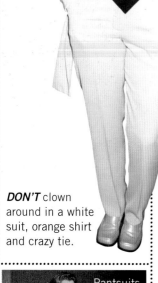

DON'T clown around in a white suit, orange shirt and crazy tie.

DO
go for the modern power suit: fitted and feminine, yet all business.

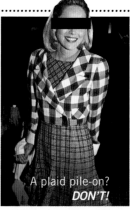

GLAMOUR FACT: IN 2004, HEIDI KLUM'S LEGS WERE INSURED FOR MORE THAN $2 MILLION.

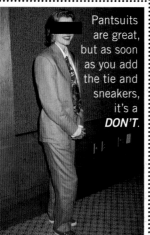

Pantsuits are great, but as soon as you add the tie and sneakers, it's a **DON'T**.

DON'T wear so many colors at once!

DO try a girly color and a flirty skirt.

A plaid pile-on? **DON'T!**

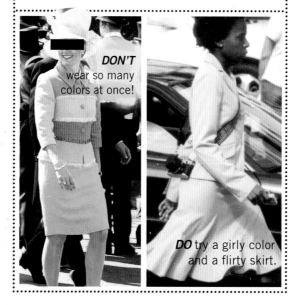

DO show style in a dark-color tweed.

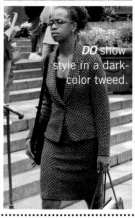

LONG JACKETS
CAN BE TRICKY

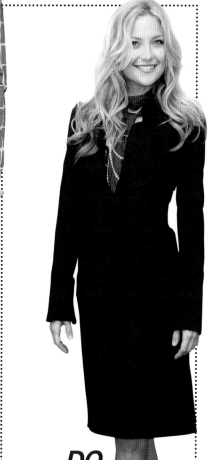

THE FITTED BLACK SUIT
A DO THEN AND NOW

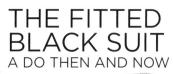

JUST DON'T!

SUITS *SEEM* SO SIMPLE. IF ONLY THEY WERE!

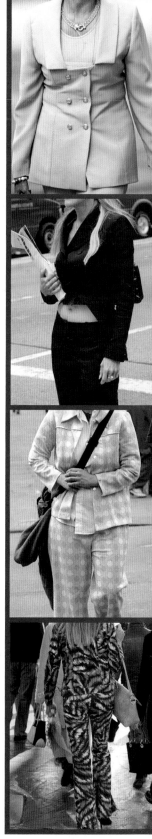

DON'T
get swallowed by a too-long, too-loud coat. (And white tights? Please, no!)

DO
try a bright blouse underneath.

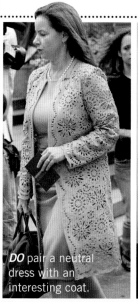

DO pair a neutral dress with an interesting coat.

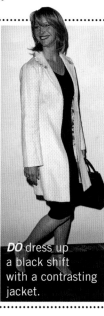

DO dress up a black shift with a contrasting jacket.

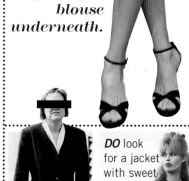

Too-big skirt and jacket? Loafers? **DON'T.**

DO look for a jacket with sweet trim like Brigitte Bardot's in 1962.

97

COATS

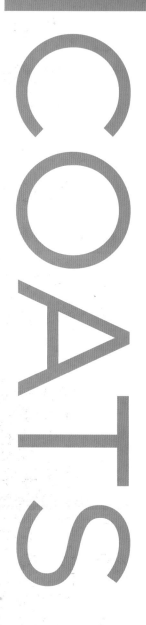

YOUR THREE BEST COATS FOR WORK

Sure, it keeps you warm (or it should), but your coat is also a major style statement, offering coworkers (and interviewers) an instant first impression. Basic colors like black, navy and camel are never-fail options, but if your work clothes tend to be neutral, liven 'em up by topping them with a fun color or pattern.

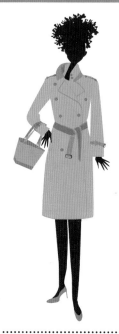

TRENCH COAT

- Look for a knee-length style that's cut slim on top—no danger of looking mannish.

- Draw attention to your waist by knotting the belt loosely. Properly tying or buckling it looks too stiff.

- Don't feel compelled to go for basic beige; bright colors are girly—and cheery on a rainy day.

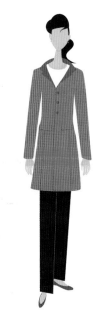

WOOL COAT

- With thicker fabrics, make sure you can fold your arms comfortably in front of you.

- Choose one that ends at the knee or just below; ankle-length styles overwhelm all but the tallest of us.

- Find a coat that is roomy enough to fit a thick sweater underneath, but fitted enough to still look tailored in warmer weather.

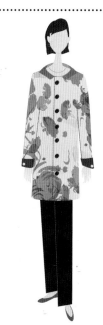

SPRING COAT

- Play around with graphic prints. A patterned spring coat is a refreshing antidote to the winter-wardrobe blahs.

- Go for a coat that's no longer than knee-length—anything floor-skimming looks mumsy.

- Make sure it's lined. Thin spring fabrics can show every bump of the clothes underneath.

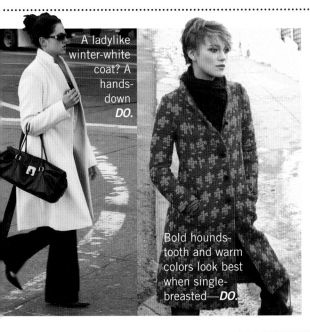

DO add style to a staple with a splash of lipstick red.

DO know you can belt an unbuttoned trench.

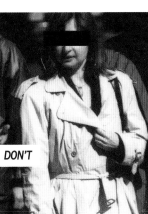

DON'T

DON'T bulk up in an overly gathered trench.

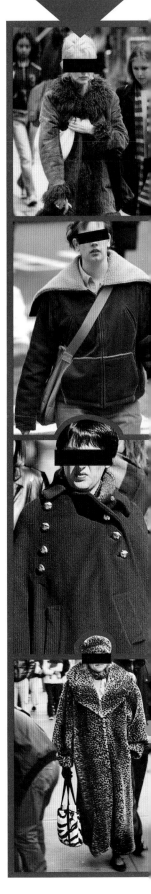

A ladylike winter-white coat? A hands-down **DO.**

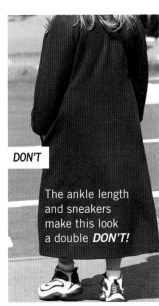

Bold houndstooth and warm colors look best when single-breasted—**DO.**

DON'T

The ankle length and sneakers make this look a double **DON'T!**

A tailored coat in a graphic print is a **DO.**

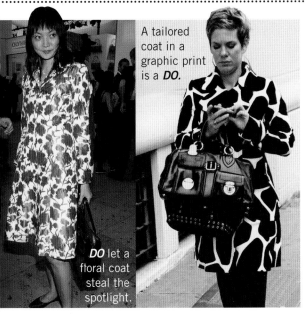

DO let a floral coat steal the spotlight.

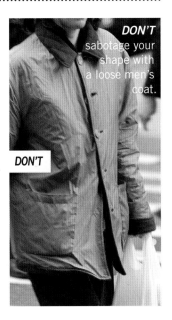

DON'T sabotage your shape with a loose men's coat.

DON'T

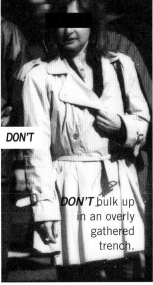

SHOES

THE ONLY WORK SHOES THAT YOU'LL NEED

They're the three classic shapes, highly versatile and—in a lively color—capable of new-ifying any outfit in your closet.

HEELS

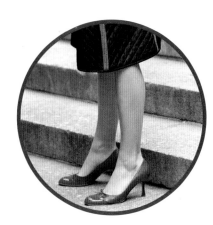

- Unless you love skyscraper heels (and can walk in them without wiping out), look for shoes in the two- to three-inch range. They lengthen legs just enough.

- For further comfort, go for heels that have rounded toes.

- Never wear strappy stiletto sandals to work; they're just too sexy for day.

FLATS

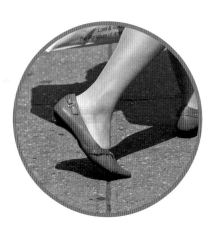

- Choose chic, ballet slipper styles in leather or fabric. Patent leather is a great dressy option.

- Leather flats can stretch out and look sloppy. Buy them in the narrowest width that fits.

- Pointed-toe styles elongate legs, but they can pinch—go for a half size longer than usual.

BOOTS

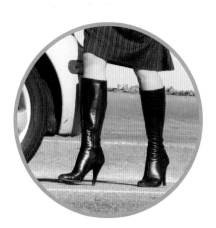

- Choose boots that go up to the bottom of your kneecaps; midcalf boots are not as professional-looking.

- Reserve your Uggs or fleece boots for snowy weekends.

- When in doubt, wear tights that are the same color as your boots—or your skirt.

DO know that every working woman needs one pair of great black heels. Or three.

DO wake up a plain outfit with a patterned heel.

DON'T choose chunky shoes—they don't flatter.

DON'T

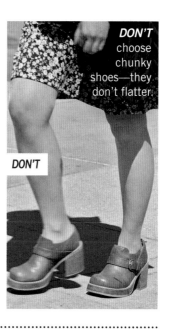

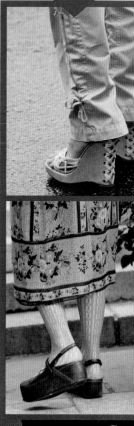

Suede loafers in a bright color are perfect for casual Fridays—*DO.*

DO add color and comfort to your day with aqua flats.

DON'T

DON'T wear your walking shoes with ankle socks to work!

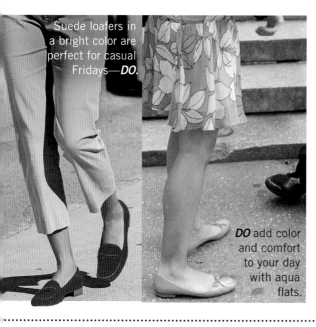

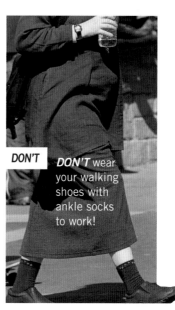

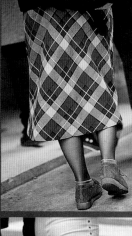

DO choose a narrow-heeled boot for a dressier look.

DO go for stacked heels if you're on your feet all day.

DON'T ever wear your go-go boots to work (unless you're a go-go dancer).

DON'T

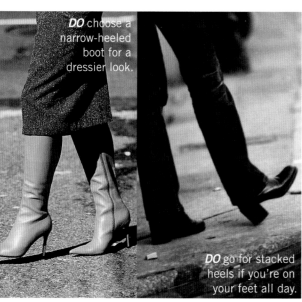

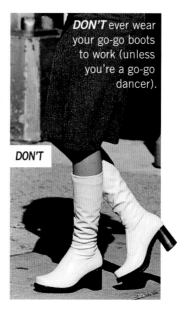

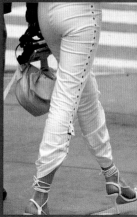

101

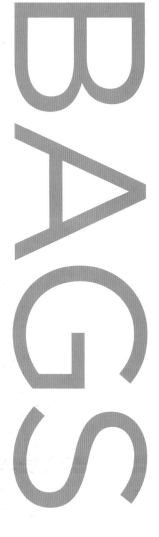

BAGS

WHICH WORK BAG DO YOU NEED?

Your bag should be able to fit all of your necessities—makeup, files, going-out shoes for later that evening—without bulging or straining. Choose bags in sync with *your* size: Petite? Keep your bag smallish, or it will dwarf you. Plus-size? Avoid those super-tiny mini clutches.

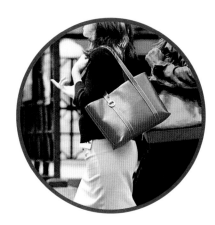

TOTE BAG

- Look for a structured shape, preferably in leather. If you go with fabric, make sure it has a flat bottom to help it hold its form.

- There's nothing more annoying than a handle that doesn't fit comfortably over your shoulder. Test it with your coat!

- Avoid totes that are heavy even when empty; you don't need to carry any extra weight.

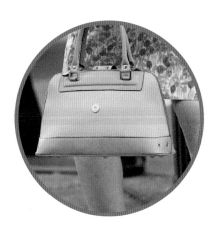

HANDBAG

- Try to get one that has a secure closure like a buckle, zipper or magnetic snap.

- If you want the look of leather, invest in the real thing; anything fake will look it.

- Only buying one? Brown is actually more versatile than black—see our DOs!

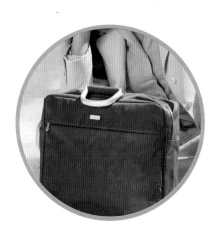

COMPUTER BAG

- Look for a structured shape with extra padding to protect your precious cargo.

- Go with a bag in a lightweight fabric or leather—your laptop's heavy enough as is.

- Make sure the strap is padded, so your hands and shoulders don't hurt.

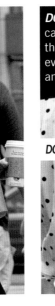

Leather trim and handles? These details are a **DO.**

DO choose a sleek, sophisticated shape.

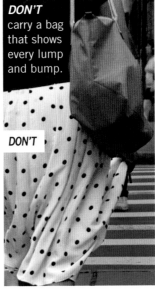

DON'T carry a bag that shows every lump and bump.

DON'T

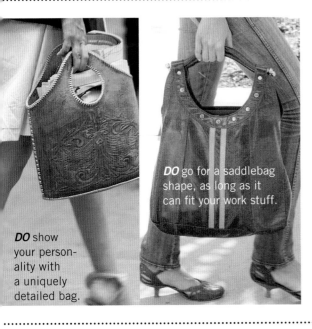

DO show your personality with a uniquely detailed bag.

DO go for a saddlebag shape, as long as it can fit your work stuff.

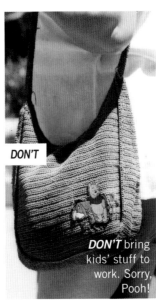

DON'T

DON'T bring kids' stuff to work. Sorry, Pooh!

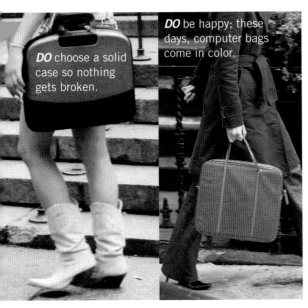

DO choose a solid case so nothing gets broken.

DO be happy; these days, computer bags come in color.

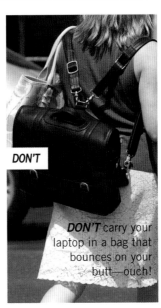

DON'T

DON'T carry your laptop in a bag that bounces on your butt—ouch!

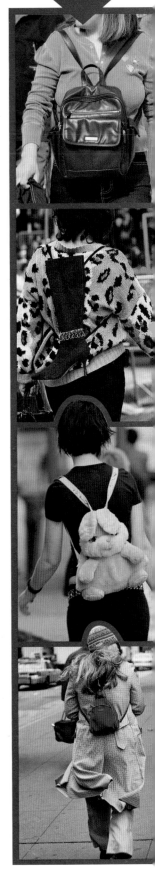

HAIR

HOW TO WEAR YOUR HAIR TO WORK

Some of the old rules, thank goodness, have finally died—now ponytails, cornrows and other "casual" styles are office-appropriate. But work hair *should* always look groomed, so watch for major messiness and anything that hangs in your face. Your hair should never eclipse *you.*

SHORT

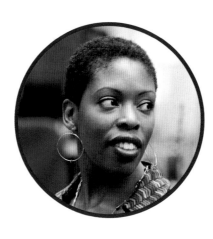

- Commit to maintaining your style with trims every six weeks.

- Choose a cut that works with your hair texture (very curly can look good extra short).

- Keep hair in place by using styling products like pomade.

- Avoid hair accessories like tiny barrettes: They'll make you look too young.

MEDIUM

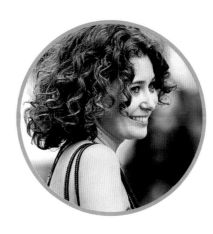

- Balance a long face with bangs or layers.

- If your hair is curly, make sure your cut looks great when straightened, too; you may want to blow it out occasionally.

- The best ponytail holder: a hair-color elastic (save the scrunchies for face-washing time).

LONG

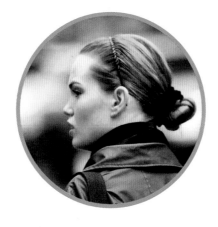

- Keep it out of your face a few different ways: Wear it half up, in a low ponytail or held back by a headband or barrettes.

- If you have thinner hair, go for long layers; they'll add movement and keep hair (and your overall look) from drooping.

- If you have a round face, consider growing your hair out—it'll visually slim your face.

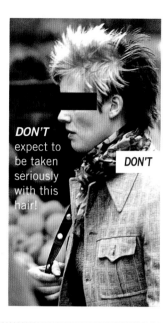

A short wispy cut shows off fine features—**DO.**

DO tuck short pieces behind your ear.

DON'T expect to be taken seriously with this hair!

DON'T

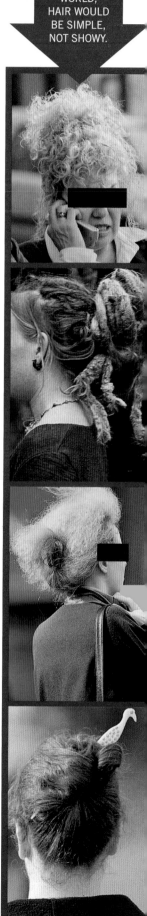

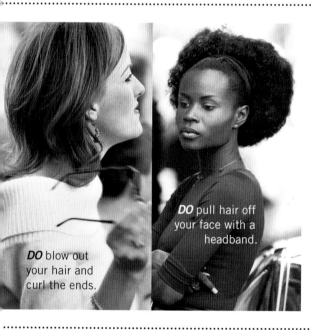

DO blow out your hair and curl the ends.

DO pull hair off your face with a headband.

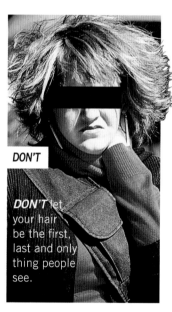

DON'T

DON'T let your hair be the first, last and only thing people see.

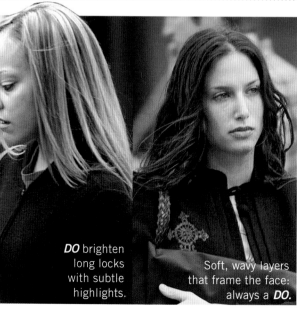

DO brighten long locks with subtle highlights.

Soft, wavy layers that frame the face: always a **DO.**

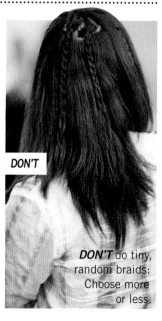

DON'T

DON'T do tiny, random braids: Choose more or less.

105

YOU'RE READY TO
ASK FOR A RAISE

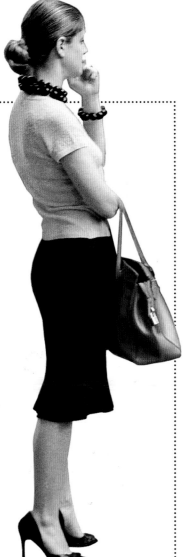

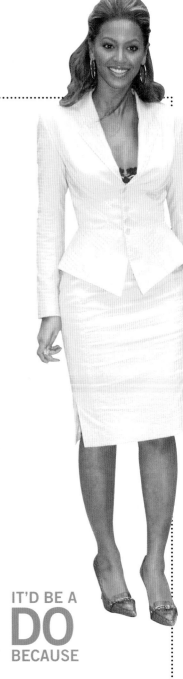

IT'D BE A
DO
BECAUSE

- A fitted blazer and top in the same color always looks great.
- The knee-length skirt and slingbacks are grown-up and chic.
- Putting hair up guarantees no nervous fiddling.

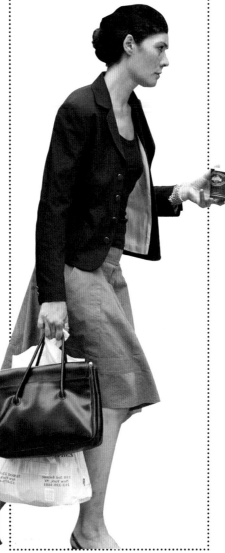

IT'D BE A
DO
BECAUSE

- Her outfit's classic and the bold jewelry shows personality.
- A fitted, flared skirt is sleek but not too sexy for work.
- A luxe leather tote shows she takes her job seriously.

IT'D BE A
DO
BECAUSE

- The bright color projects a positive, take-charge attitude.
- Pulling back long hair keeps it professional.
- The skirt's not too short. Beyoncé, you've got the raise!

YOU'VE EARNED IT. YOU DESERVE IT. Get yourself ready to face your boss and ask for it by stepping up to the plate, stylewise. Your goal: to look as mature and confident as you feel. Your outfit should make you look like the top-of-the-line teacher, salesperson or executive that you are. So break out the iron, sew a falling hem and, most important, choose a *polished* outfit that makes you feel like you could rule the world. Because you could be just a few raises away from doing just that!

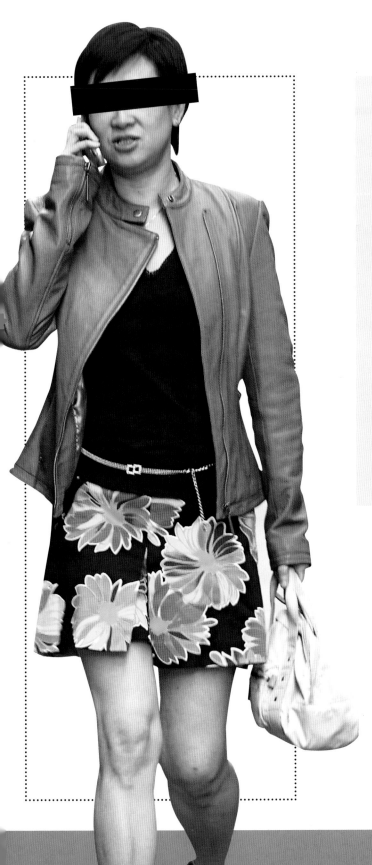

Five Investment Pieces

...TO ACQUIRE *AFTER* YOU GET YOUR RAISE

1.
A perfect suit
Spring for the triple threat: jacket, skirt *and* pants, and wear them separately too.

2.
A great work bag
Big enough to cart home papers, small enough to not look schleppy for after-work drinks.

3.
A fitted trench coat

4.
A fancy watch
(Save the digital one for the gym.)

5.
A pair of fabulous heels

IT'D BE A
DON'T
BECAUSE

- Skirts this short at work are always risky. Why sabotage an important day? (If she's off to the beach, though, she's fine!)
- A loud print distracts from the issue at hand: your career and salary.
- Too-long jacket sleeves complete the too-young impression.

IT'S CASUAL FRIDAY

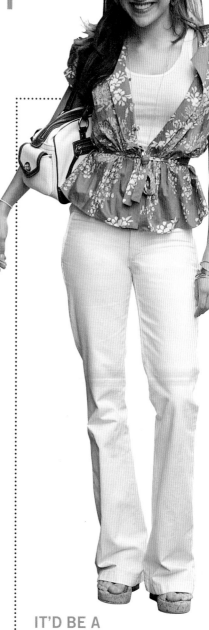

IT'D BE A
DO
BECAUSE

- Her long shorts are cool yet work-appropriate.
- A sleek vest over an untucked, fitted shirt could be your new Friday uniform.
- The bold watch is a great accent (and shows she's still on the clock).

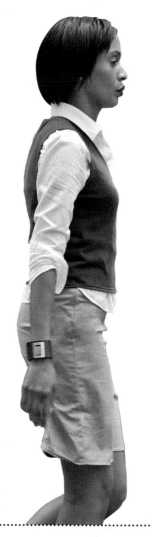

IT'D BE A
DO
BECAUSE

- The fitted top and full skirt prevent her from showing too much skin.
- Her bag and slides are both in professional black.
- Her outfit is in always-right neutral colors.

IT'D BE A
DO
BECAUSE

- Over a tank, a floral blouse acts like a casual jacket.
- White trousers are a perfect alternative to black or brown.
- Cork platforms and gold jewelry offer the perfect finishing touches.

ALTHOUGH CASUAL FRIDAY IS THE ONE DAY OF THE WEEK when you're actually invited to dress down, it's a bit of a phony invitation: Your boss doesn't *really* want you casual, alas. Work, after all, is still work. To loosen up and still impress your superiors, sub flats for heels, pressed khakis or jeans for a skirt, or a nice T-shirt for a blouse. And think about trying out a new style idea or two, like wearing loads of jewelry with a vintage blouse or colorful wedge espadrilles with long shorts. But keep playing it safe with your hair and makeup (purple eyeliner is for weekends only).

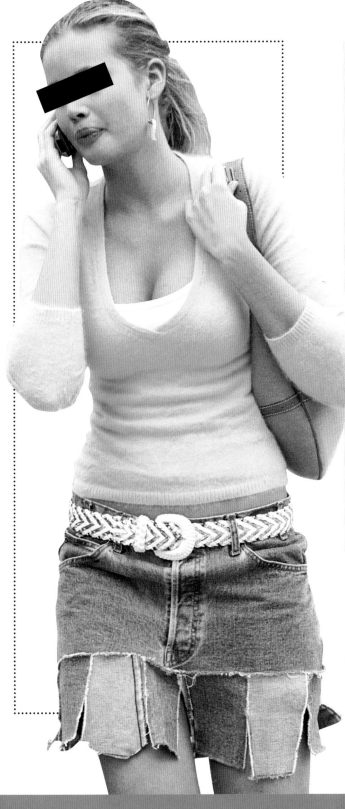

Four Things You Should Never, Ever Wear to Work
(EVEN ON FRIDAYS)

1.
Tube tops
Only appropriate for small children.

2.
Cheeky message tees
A shirt that says "Gettin' lucky in Kentucky" will never win you a raise or respect. So DON'T.

3.
Cutoffs
Daisy Dukes are a no-brainer no-no, but jeans you've "hemmed" by trimming off the excess length and letting the ends fray also have no place at work.

4.
Sweatpants
Because, as Jerry once said to George on *Seinfeld*, "You know the message you're sending out to the world with these sweatpants? You're telling the world, 'I give up.'"

IT'D BE A
DON'T
BECAUSE

- Cleavage? OK for downtime— but not great if she's going to work.
- The cut-up denim skirt says "I'm off to the beach," not "I'm worth every buck you pay me."

IS IT A DO OR A DON'T?

Even if you're strong enough to lug your worldly goods, DON'T!

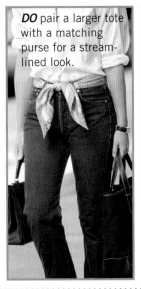

DO pair a pretty dress with flip-flops for casual moments.

FLIP-FLOPS

In the steamy months, stuffing your feet into regular shoes feels like torture. Flip-flops are a perfect commuter solution—just change once you get to your desk.

OUR VERDICT:
usually a DO

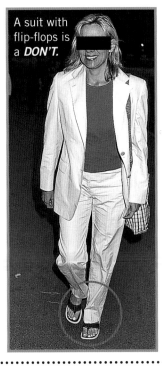

A suit with flip-flops is a **DON'T.**

MULTIPLE BAGS

Carting around everything you need for work (and after) is a necessary evil. But rather than being a DON'T with two giant totes, pare down possessions to the essentials—and put gym clothes in a separate bag.

OUR VERDICT:
a DO (if done right)

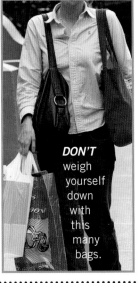

DO pair a larger tote with a matching purse for a streamlined look.

DON'T weigh yourself down with this many bags.

THE SCHOOLGIRL LOOK

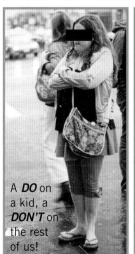

A **DO** on a kid, a **DON'T** on the rest of us!

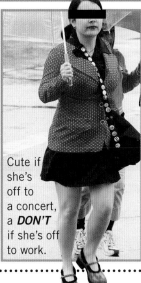

Cute if she's off to a concert, a **DON'T** if she's off to work.

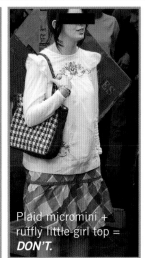

Plaid micromini + ruffly little-girl top = **DON'T.**

The schoolgirl look (think Kelly Osbourne in those short plaid skirts) can be cute and flirty in certain venues, but do you really want your boss to think of you that way? No. If you can't resist a little-girl touch, be sure that the rest of your clothing is ultra-professional.

OUR VERDICT:
a definite DON'T

CLEAVAGE

Cleavage is wonderful. Cleavage is fabulous. Cleavage is sexy—too sexy for work. When in doubt, cover up for the office.

OUR VERDICT:
a DON'T at work

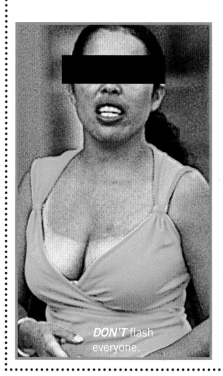

DON'T flash everyone.

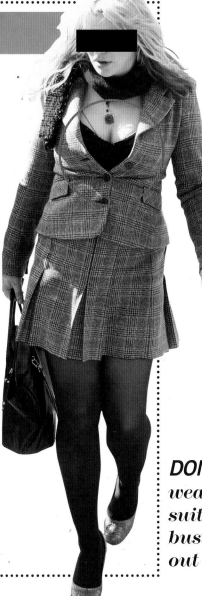

DON'T *wear a suit you're busting out of!*

ALWAYS **A DON'T** AT WORK

Sequins, sparkles or spangles as more than an accent

Baseball hats

Floor-length skirts

Bustiers

Dirty sneakers

Microminis

Skintight anything

Six-inch nails

Visible belly rings

Pleather

Multiple exposed tattoos

"I NEED
TO LOOK LIKE
A PROFESSIONAL!"

With plans to start her own bakery, Samiyyah needs to look more like a business owner and less like a student. "This sweater and skirt [below] are from my college days," she says. Solution: take-charge outfits that fit her energetic personality. The rules of grown-up dress-up for her (and you) to follow? Fitted shapes (nothing oversize!), *adult* patterns (sorry, no Fair Isle stripes) and heels whenever possible.

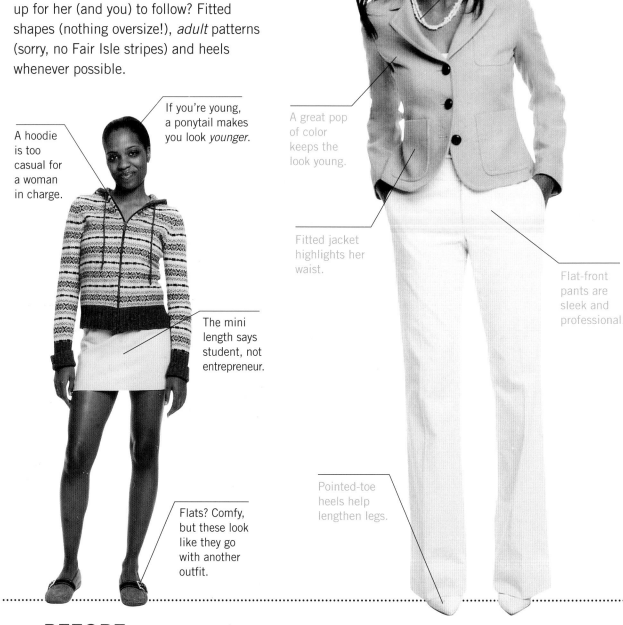

Neutral lipstick isn't over-powering.

Necklace adds a polished touch.

A great pop of color keeps the look young.

Fitted jacket highlights her waist.

Flat-front pants are sleek and professional.

If you're young, a ponytail makes you look *younger*.

A hoodie is too casual for a woman in charge.

The mini length says student, not entrepreneur.

Flats? Comfy, but these look like they go with another outfit.

Pointed-toe heels help lengthen legs.

BEFORE:
Samiyyah Williams, 23

THE BIG MEETING

"It's comfortable but professional. And it definitely reflects my personal style."

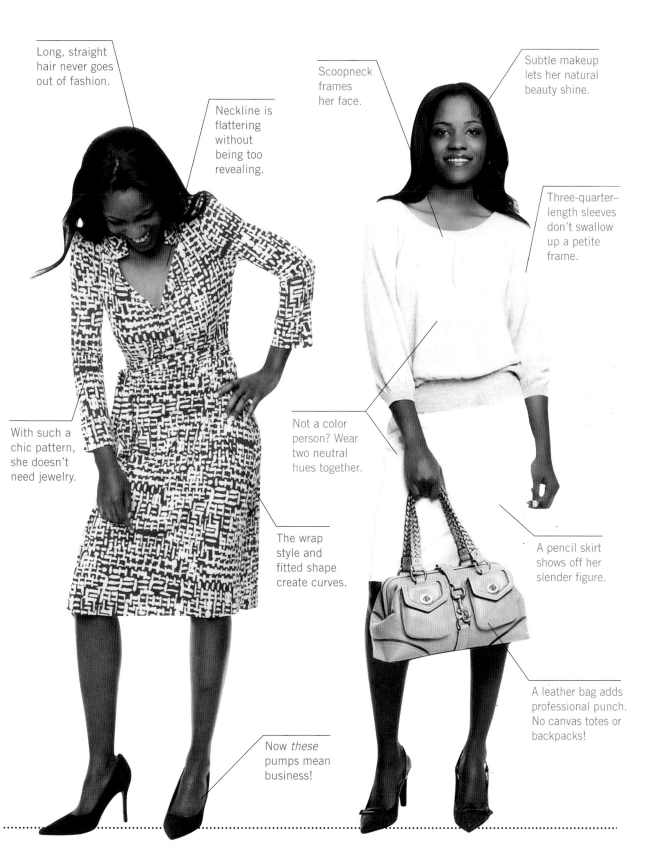

Long, straight hair never goes out of fashion.

Neckline is flattering without being too revealing.

Scoopneck frames her face.

Subtle makeup lets her natural beauty shine.

Three-quarter–length sleeves don't swallow up a petite frame.

With such a chic pattern, she doesn't need jewelry.

Not a color person? Wear two neutral hues together.

The wrap style and fitted shape create curves.

A pencil skirt shows off her slender figure.

A leather bag adds professional punch. No canvas totes or backpacks!

Now *these* pumps mean business!

FIRST DAY AT WORK

"This gives my body curves, and I love how fun it is."

CLIENT LUNCH

"Such a flexible outfit! In a flash, I can dress it up or down."

"I NEED
WORK CLOTHES
I CAN GO OUT IN!"

As a personal assistant to a high-powered boss, Adriana is often the go-to after-hours hostess for her organization—a job she's underdressed for in the outfit below. "I bought it when I was looking for basic officewear," she says. But in this case, what she ended up with were unflattering shapes in shades of blah. So what *do* you wear for work evenings? Here, chic choices that help Adriana look like the key player she is.

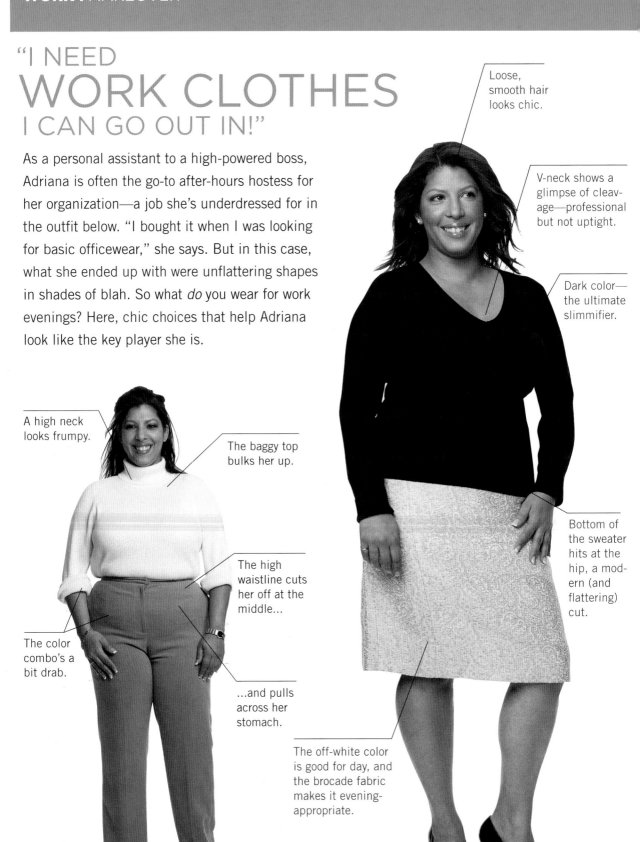

Loose, smooth hair looks chic.

V-neck shows a glimpse of cleavage—professional but not uptight.

Dark color—the ultimate slimmifier.

A high neck looks frumpy.

The baggy top bulks her up.

The high waistline cuts her off at the middle...

The color combo's a bit drab.

...and pulls across her stomach.

Bottom of the sweater hits at the hip, a modern (and flattering) cut.

The off-white color is good for day, and the brocade fabric makes it evening-appropriate.

BEFORE:
Adriana Martinez, 36

OFFICE PARTY

"I always have problems finding tops that fit my chest. This covers me *and* looks fantastic!"

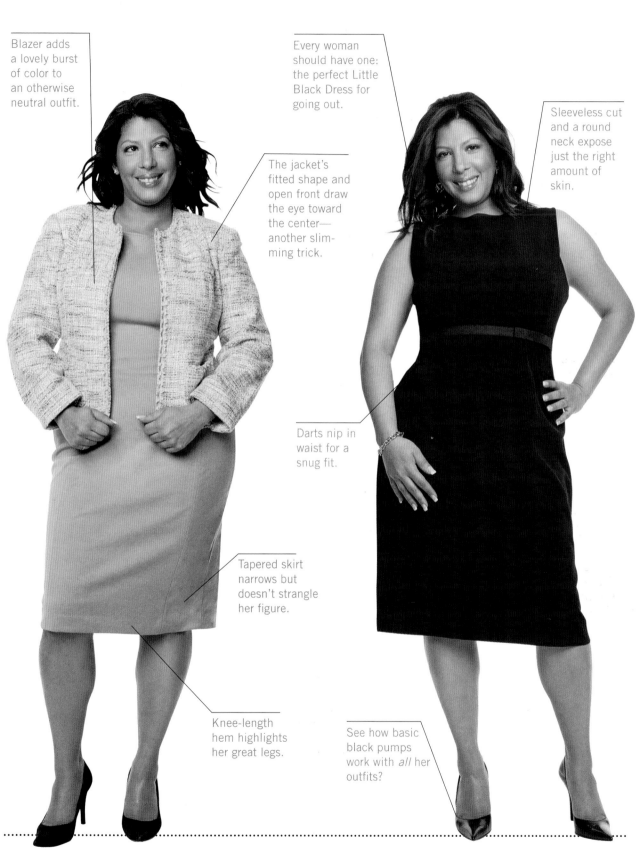

Blazer adds a lovely burst of color to an otherwise neutral outfit.

Every woman should have one: the perfect Little Black Dress for going out.

The jacket's fitted shape and open front draw the eye toward the center— another slimming trick.

Sleeveless cut and a round neck expose just the right amount of skin.

Darts nip in waist for a snug fit.

Tapered skirt narrows but doesn't strangle her figure.

Knee-length hem highlights her great legs.

See how basic black pumps work with *all* her outfits?

AFTER-WORK DRINKS

"Perfect for cocktails; this can easily go from day to night."

DINNER WITH CLIENTS

"This makes my curves look great—and it's perfect for the business dinners we host all around the world."

"I'VE GOT THE BIG JOB—NOW I NEED THE RIGHT CLOTHES!"

This new mom just returned to a top-level job as an advertising account director but was in desperate need of a wardrobe update. "I've had this shirt for years, and my mother made me buy these pants ages ago," Jennifer says. Here, she's shown in bright colors and stylish shapes that fit her dynamic personality *and* big job.

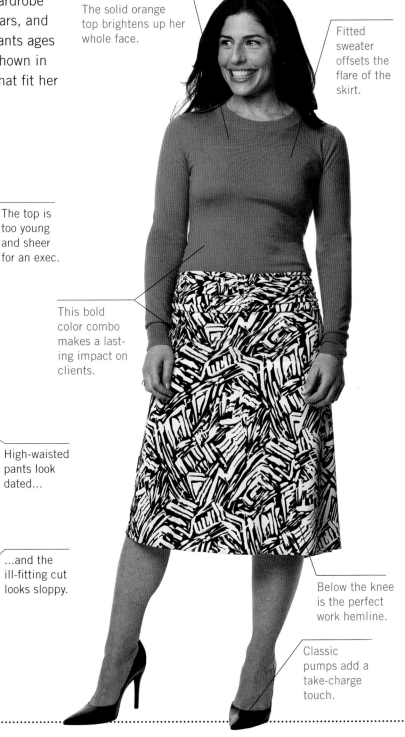

The solid orange top brightens up her whole face.

Fitted sweater offsets the flare of the skirt.

The muddy colors and patterns wash her out.

The top is too young and sheer for an exec.

This bold color combo makes a lasting impact on clients.

High-waisted pants look dated...

...and the ill-fitting cut looks sloppy.

Below the knee is the perfect work hemline.

Classic pumps add a take-charge touch.

BEFORE:
Jennifer Schwab, 34

EVERY DAY AT THE OFFICE
"This colorful outfit gives me confidence and totally reflects my personality, as opposed to standard black pants and a plain sweater."

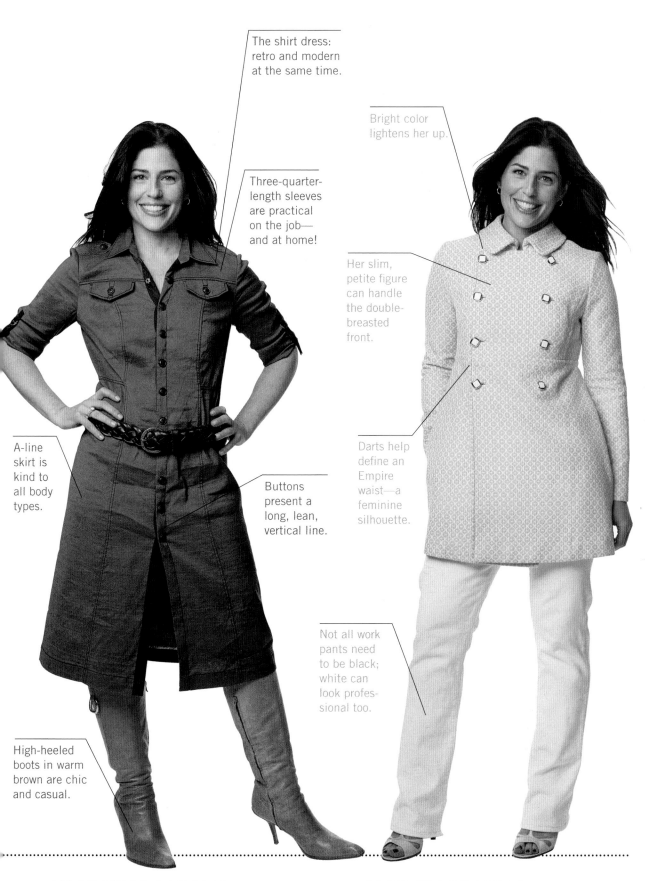

The shirt dress: retro and modern at the same time.

Three-quarter-length sleeves are practical on the job— and at home!

Bright color lightens her up.

Her slim, petite figure can handle the double-breasted front.

A-line skirt is kind to all body types.

Buttons present a long, lean, vertical line.

Darts help define an Empire waist—a feminine silhouette.

Not all work pants need to be black; white can look professional too.

High-heeled boots in warm brown are chic and casual.

WORKING LUNCH

"This looks smart—and that's how you want to look when you're trying to impress a new client."

CLIENT MEETING

"This is so much more fun than a suit! It says I don't take myself too seriously, so it's great for a more social event like lunch."

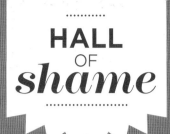

HALL OF *shame*

ULTIMATE DENIM DON'TS!
THEY'RE EVERYWHERE: SCARY LOW RISES, EXTREME ACID WASH AND WORSE!

Elvis lives on in airbrushed glory! ***DON'T.***

If you need a bikini wax to wear it, it's a ***DON'T.***

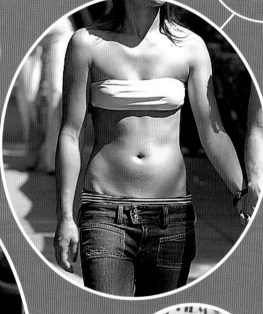

What's with the weird bleach? These are a ***DON'T.***

DON'T wear the scratching-post look!

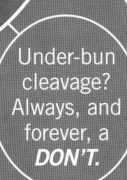

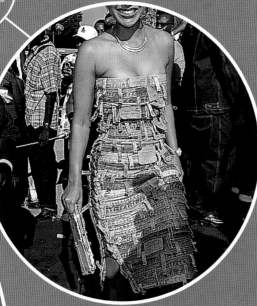

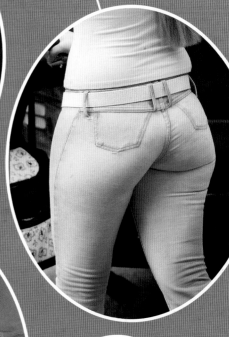

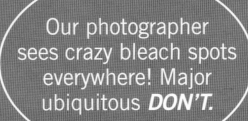

DON'T you wonder why anyone ever thought this was a good idea?

DON'T neglect fit. This hurts just looking at it.

Under-bun cleavage? Always, and forever, a **DON'T.**

Our photographer sees crazy bleach spots everywhere! Major ubiquitous **DON'T.**

Denim leg warmers?!?! Umm, **DON'T.**

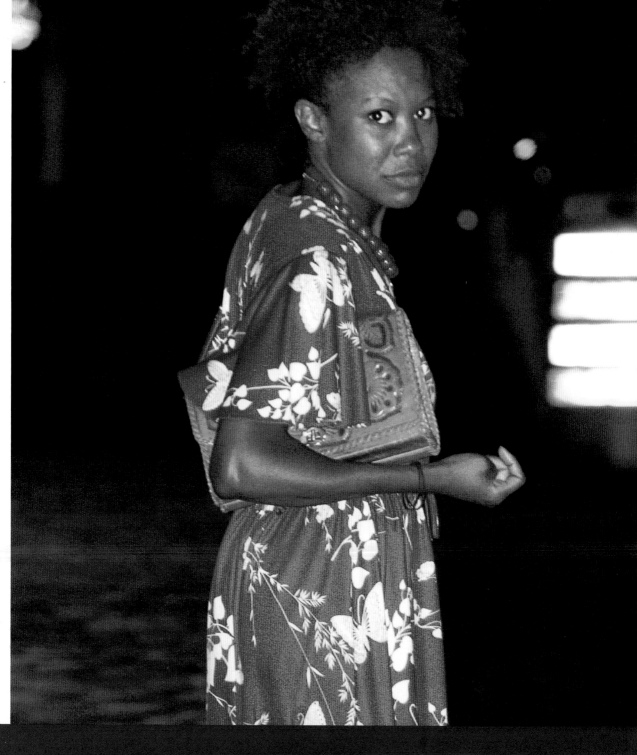

YOUR

DO

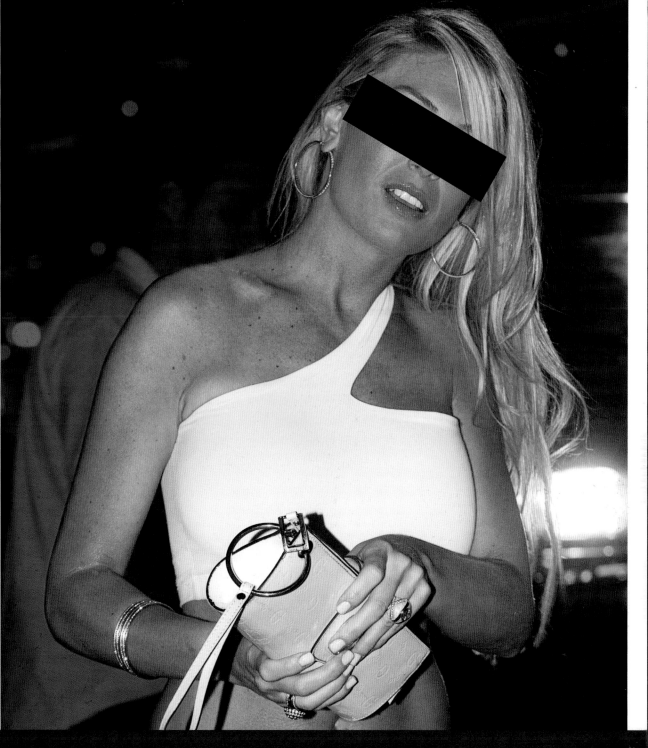

NIGHTS OUT

WHAT WORKS IN YOUR WORLD AFTER DARK

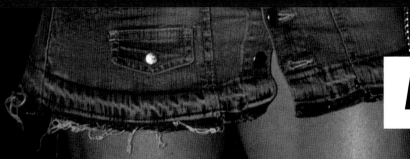

DON'T

THE RULES

for night

DON'T SHOW
EVERYTHING ALL AT ONCE.

*While flashing some skin is sexy, stick to exposing just
one area. Choose either a slit skirt or a cleavage-baring top,
for instance, but not both at the same time.*

EMBRACE THE POWER OF HEELS.

*Even a little wedge or kitten heel lengthens your legs
and can make you feel more powerful, seductive and feminine.
What's not to love?*

REMEMBER, "SEXY"
DOESN'T MEAN "SKINTIGHT."

*Dressing for after dark means that you can be a little
more daring, but painted-on clothes are always unflattering.
(Besides, it's nice to be able to breathe.) A simple rule: If you
wear one curve-hugging piece, pair it with a fuller one.*

GET YOURSELF SOME CUTE,
BARE-ISH TOPS.

*They're the foundation of your going-out wardrobe.
Add jeans or a black skirt, a jacket or sweater, heels, jewelry—
maybe a cap or scarf—and you're set for everything
from dates to girls' nights to birthday dinners.*

GO WITH JUST A TOUCH OF SHIMMER.

Sequins and glitzy details are fun and festive when they gleam from a single item like a top or an accessory like a belt. But squelch any impulse to shine all over, or you'll be heading into Vegas showgirl territory.

 IF YOU CAN FOLLOW ONLY ONE RULE, THIS IS IT!

WHEN YOU FIND THE PERFECT LITTLE BLACK DRESS, GRAB IT.

Even if it's at the higher end of your price range, spring for it. That LBD will be worth every penny—you'll dress it up and down for years to come.

BE ON THE LOOKOUT FOR FLATTERING BLACK PANTS, TOO.

Another item that's nighttime gold—get two pairs if you can.

LEAVE YOUR WORK PURSE AT WORK.

Same goes for your laptop or gym tote; a workhorse of a bag is cumbersome and annoying. Keep a little clutch in your big bag, pop it out and check your albatross at the door.

BRING ON THE HAIRSPRAY AND ACCESSORIES!

Even women with beautiful hair find it looking less than perfect after a day of work. So if you have a post-5 P.M. event, make sure you have what you need to revive your 'do—keep a stash in a drawer.

OWN ONE GREAT PAIR OF NIGHTTIME EARRINGS THAT YOU'D NEVER WEAR DURING THE DAY.

They're brilliant for making an impression at a dinner or a bar, places where you'll be seen mainly from the waist up.

TOPS

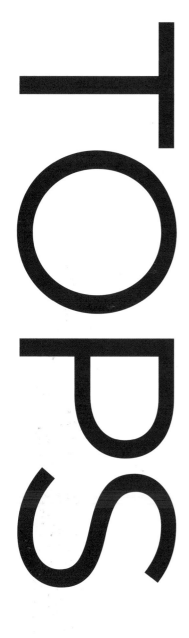

THREE TOPS FOR EVENING

Nighttime is perfect for showcasing your sexy back, toned shoulders, graceful neck or seductive cleavage. But avoid overexposure: Pick tops that highlight just one or two zones.

❶ TUNIC

- Choose a flared style that's fitted at the shoulders *and* under the bust so that you don't look pregnant (unless you are, of course).

- Look for a V-neck for a sexier edge.

- Pair with straight-cut, slim-fit pants to balance the top's fullness.

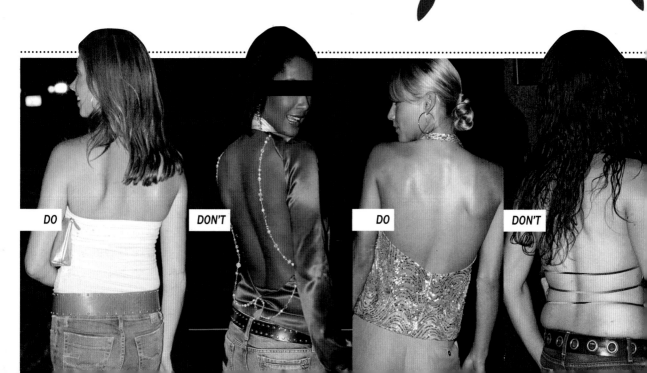

DO   DON'T   DO   DON'T

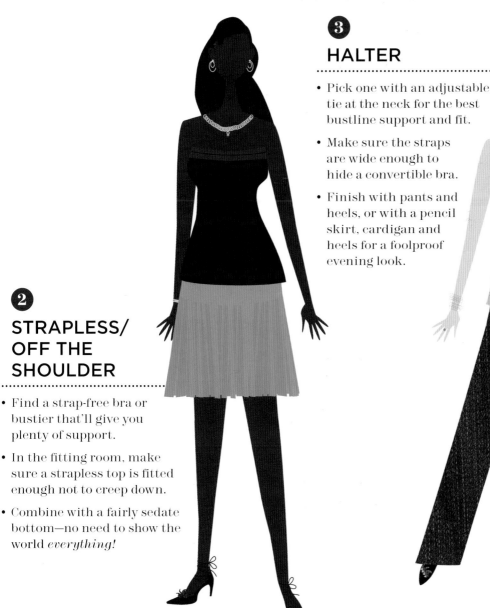

③ HALTER

- Pick one with an adjustable tie at the neck for the best bustline support and fit.
- Make sure the straps are wide enough to hide a convertible bra.
- Finish with pants and heels, or with a pencil skirt, cardigan and heels for a foolproof evening look.

② STRAPLESS/ OFF THE SHOULDER

- Find a strap-free bra or bustier that'll give you plenty of support.
- In the fitting room, make sure a strapless top is fitted enough not to creep down.
- Combine with a fairly sedate bottom—no need to show the world *everything!*

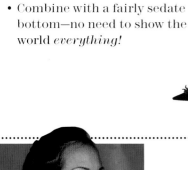

DO

Style Clinic

The DOs & DON'Ts of backless tops

You rarely see your own back, but other people *do*. Before you go backless, assess your comfort level. You can expose your shoulder blades relatively risk-free; more extreme styles, however, may look and feel more like lobster bibs than actual tops. And if your bra size is any larger than an A, definitely wear a stick-on or other invisible bra.

"Showing a woman's back is alluring without being obvious." —OSCAR DE LA RENTA, DESIGNER

THE BIG
DOS&DON'TS OF
TOPS

EVENING SHIRTS
BUTTON UP!

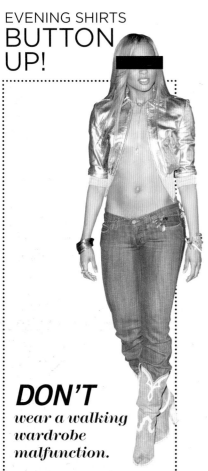

DON'T
wear a walking wardrobe malfunction.

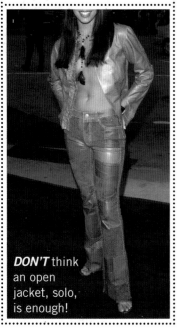

DON'T think an open jacket, solo, is enough!

THE ONE-OF-A-KIND TEE
IT'S SO YOU

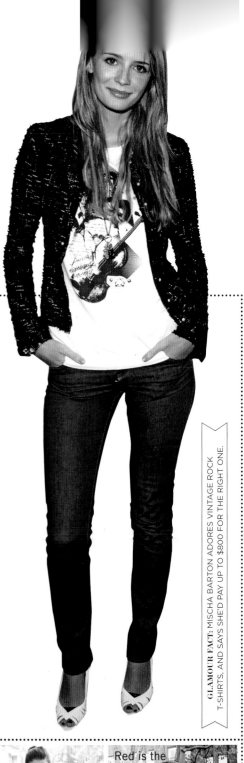

DO
mix a fancy jacket with a rocker T-shirt.

GLAMOUR FACT: MISCHA BARTON ADORES VINTAGE ROCK T-SHIRTS, AND SAYS SHE'D PAY UP TO $800 FOR THE RIGHT ONE.

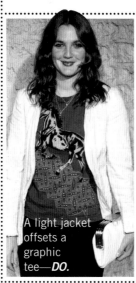

A light jacket offsets a graphic tee—**DO.**

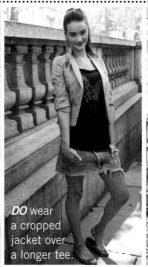

DO wear a cropped jacket over a longer tee.

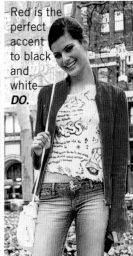

Red is the perfect accent to black and white— **DO.**

EIGHT TOPS
TO AVOID

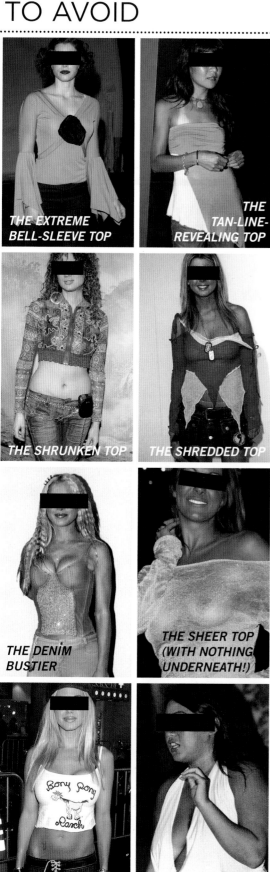

**THE EXTREME
BELL-SLEEVE TOP**

**THE
TAN-LINE-
REVEALING TOP**

THE SHRUNKEN TOP

THE SHREDDED TOP

**THE DENIM
BUSTIER**

**THE SHEER TOP
(WITH NOTHING
UNDERNEATH!)**

THE CUTOFF TANK

THE TOO-LOW TOP

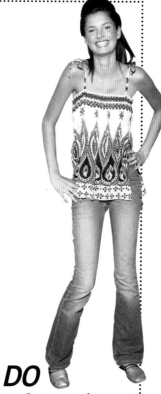

DO
*make your jeans
evening-ready
with a shoulder-
showing,
patterned top.*

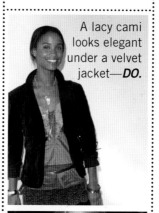

A lacy cami
looks elegant
under a velvet
jacket—**DO**.

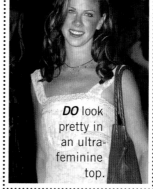

DO look
pretty in
an ultra-
feminine
top.

LET'S CALL
THESE THE
ANTI ROLE-
MODEL TOPS.

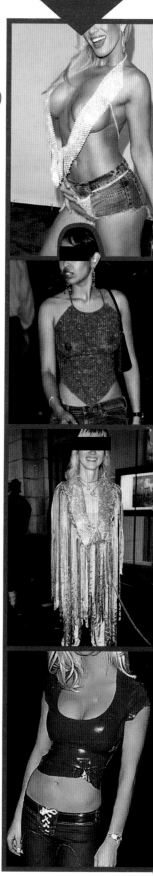

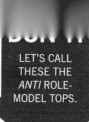

PANTS

THREE ALL-YOU-NEED EVENING PANTS

Hot date? Dinner with his family? You need a great pair of pants. Skip the baggy, pleated ones (neither flatters anything) or the hyper-trendy; get a flat-front, straight-leg style in a dressed-up fabric like velvet or satin for your dressiest occasions—and slimmer pants and great jeans for more casual moments.

❶ TROUSERS

- Look for a straight cut or, if you're pear-shaped, a style that's a little flared from the knee. (It'll balance your hips.)

- If you're wearing a light color, make sure you don't have a peek-a-boo underwear situation.

- Wear with round- or pointed-toe heels; they'll lengthen your legs.

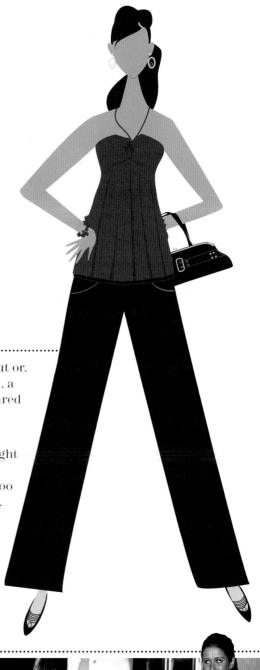

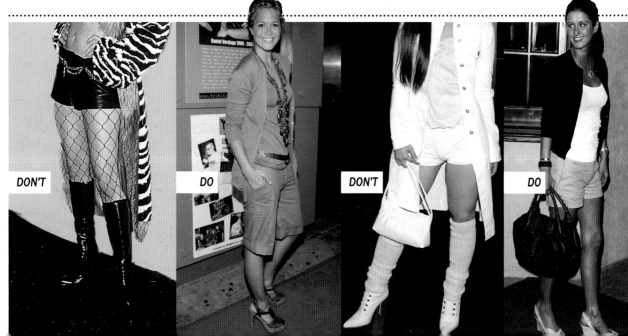

DON'T

DO

DON'T

DO

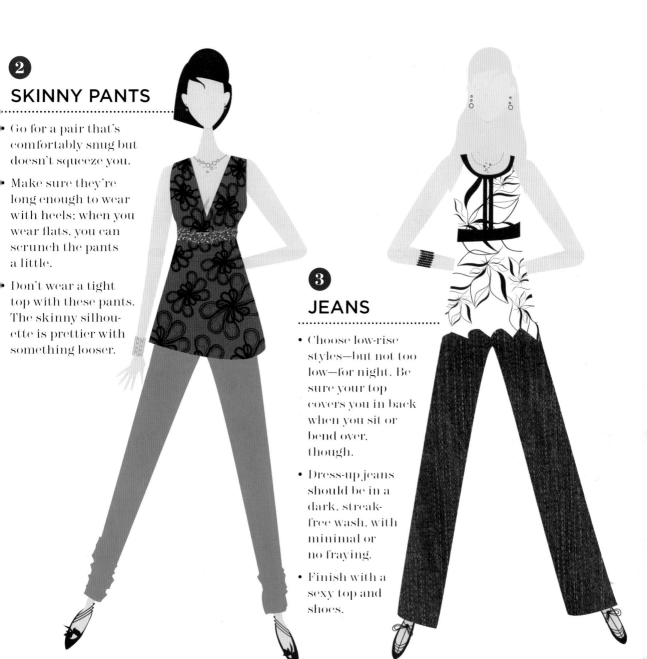

❷ SKINNY PANTS

- Go for a pair that's comfortably snug but doesn't squeeze you.

- Make sure they're long enough to wear with heels; when you wear flats, you can scrunch the pants a little.

- Don't wear a tight top with these pants. The skinny silhouette is prettier with something looser.

❸ JEANS

- Choose low-rise styles—but not too low—for night. Be sure your top covers you in back when you sit or bend over, though.

- Dress-up jeans should be in a dark, streak-free wash, with minimal or no fraying.

- Finish with a sexy top and shoes.

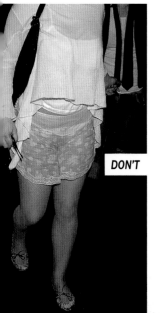

DON'T

Style Clinic

The DOs & DON'Ts of nighttime shorts

Recently, celebs have adopted this daytime favorite for evenings out on the town. Done right, P.M. shorts look chicly carefree and show off great legs. The newest styles are longer, Bermuda-length shorts that can easily be dressed up or down via your shoes and top. If you're dying to try shorter shorts, make sure that they hit at least midthigh; save anything smaller for the beach.

"A girl should be two things: classy and fabulous."
—COCO CHANEL, DESIGNER

THE BIG
DOS&DON'TS OF
PANTS

FIND THE
PERFECT LENGTH

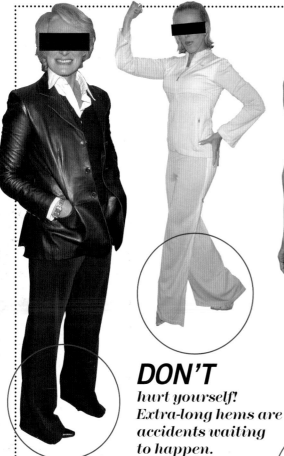

DON'T
*hurt yourself!
Extra-long hems are
accidents waiting
to happen.*

DO
*look for pants that
stop just short of the
ground. You didn't get
that pedicure for nothing!*

HOW BAGGY IS
TOO BAGGY?

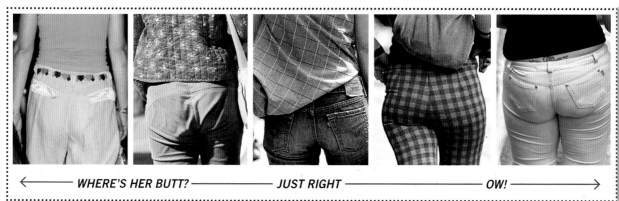

← —— WHERE'S HER BUTT? —— JUST RIGHT —— OW! →

BE A
DENIM DO

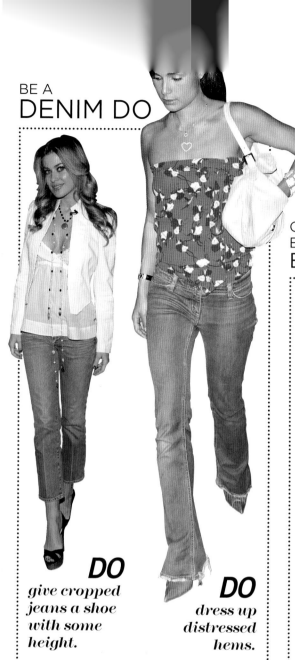

DO *give cropped jeans a shoe with some height.*

DO *dress up distressed hems.*

CROPPED PANTS: ELEGANT ENOUGH FOR EVENING

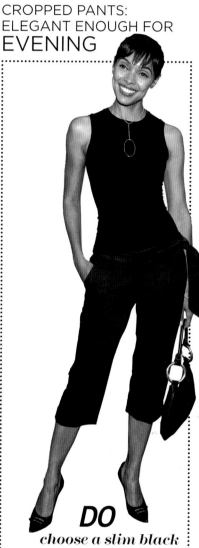

DO *choose a slim black pair for a sleek look.*

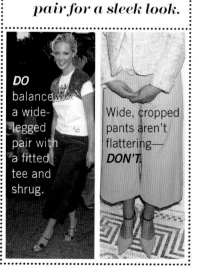

DO balance a wide-legged pair with a fitted tee and shrug.

Wide, cropped pants aren't flattering—**DON'T**.

...NOT A DON'T!

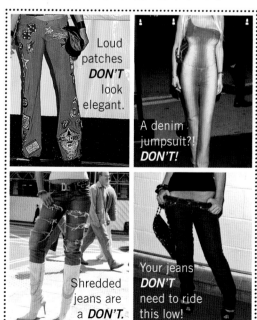

Loud patches **DON'T** look elegant.

A denim jumpsuit?! **DON'T!**

Shredded jeans are a **DON'T**.

Your jeans **DON'T** need to ride this low!

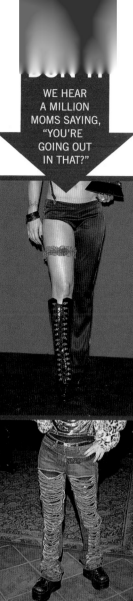

WE HEAR A MILLION MOMS SAYING, "YOU'RE GOING OUT IN THAT?"

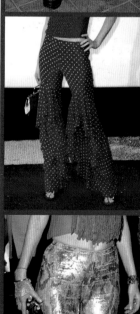

DRESSES

WHAT SHOULD I WEAR FOR DATE NIGHT?

Sometimes, only a dress will do. Basic fitting-room advice: Pick one that shows off your best feature, whether it's your alluring shoulders, curvy waist or long legs. DON'T try to highlight with both a low-cut top and short hem—too bare!

❶ FLOWY

- Find styles that are fitted on the top, not full all over.
- Wear a hemline that hits just at or below the knee—it works on most body types.
- Try styles with layers of sheer, light fabric, like chiffon, for a soft look that isn't see-through.

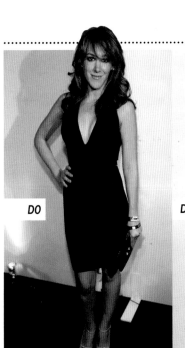

DO

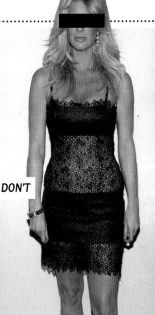

DON'T

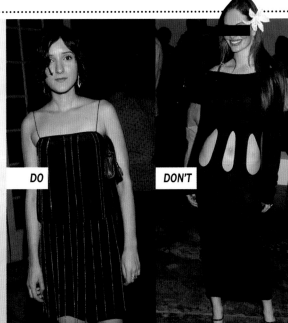

DO

DON'T

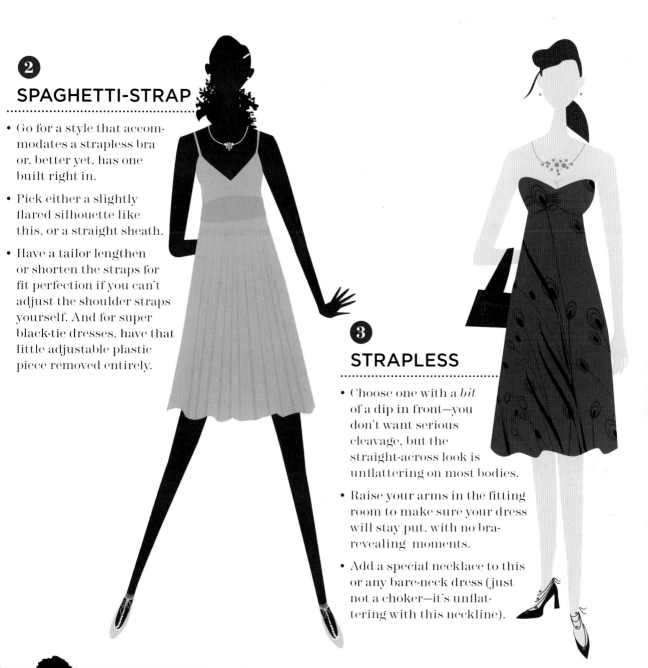

② SPAGHETTI-STRAP

- Go for a style that accommodates a strapless bra or, better yet, has one built right in.
- Pick either a slightly flared silhouette like this, or a straight sheath.
- Have a tailor lengthen or shorten the straps for fit perfection if you can't adjust the shoulder straps yourself. And for super black-tie dresses, have that little adjustable plastic piece removed entirely.

③ STRAPLESS

- Choose one with a *bit* of a dip in front—you don't want serious cleavage, but the straight-across look is unflattering on most bodies.
- Raise your arms in the fitting room to make sure your dress will stay put, with no bra-revealing moments.
- Add a special necklace to this or any bare-neck dress (just not a choker—it's unflattering with this neckline).

DO

Style Clinic

The DOs & DON'Ts of the Little Black Dress

We all know that an Audrey Hepburn–style LBD is a must-have. Dress it up or down: Top with a fitted cardigan; play with heels in varying heights and colors (yes, color's cool with black); wear with fine or groovier jewelry. Classic shapes like a sheath will have style longevity and work for whatever life might throw at you—just pass up gimmicky LBDs and you'll always be a DO.

"Fashion offers no greater challenge than finding what works for night without looking like you are wearing a costume."
—VERA WANG, DESIGNER

THE BIG
DOS&DON'TS OF
DRESSES

THE SHEER DRESS
BEWARE OF
OVEREXPOSURE!

PATTERNS
DONE
RIGHT...

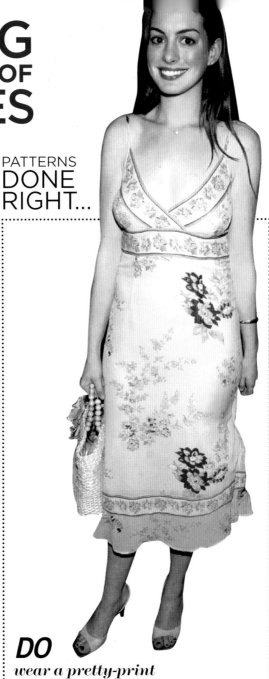

DON'T
*go braless under
a see-through
dress.*

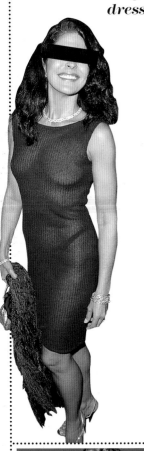

DO
*wear a pretty-print
Empire-waist dress.*

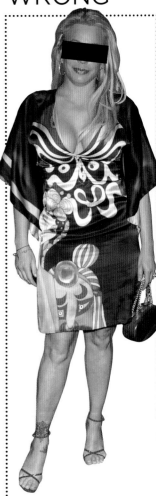

DON'T
*choose a print
that draws
attention to places
that don't need it!*

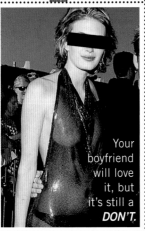

Your
boyfriend
will love
it, but
it's still a
DON'T.

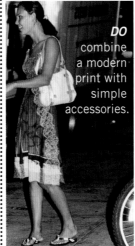

DO
combine
a modern
print with
simple
accessories.

DO offset
a busier
pattern
with a
solid
cardigan.

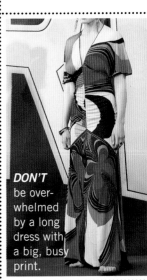

DON'T
be over-
whelmed
by a long
dress with
a big, busy
print.

BE BOLD WITH
COLOR

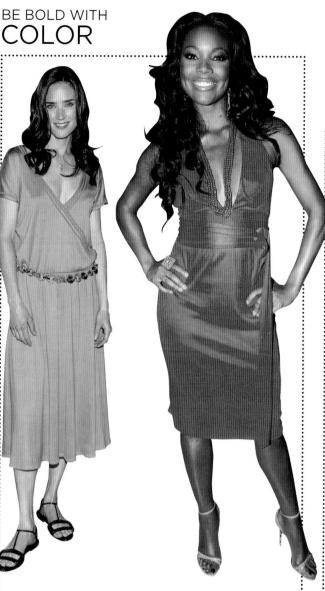

THE
OFF-THE-SHOULDER
DRESS
A DO THEN,
A DO NOW

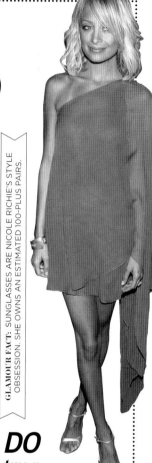

DO
keep the focus on
your dress with
neutral sandals.

DO
look va-va-voom
in eternally
sexy red.

DO
try a
shoulder-
baring style in
a look-at-me
color.

DO give your
tank dress an
extra layer of
prettiness.

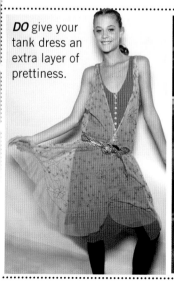

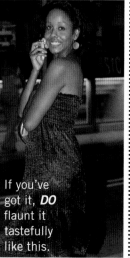

If you've
got it, *DO*
flaunt it
tastefully
like this.

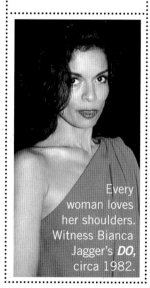

Every
woman loves
her shoulders.
Witness Bianca
Jagger's *DO*,
circa 1982.

DON'T

INDIVIDUAL
STYLE—GOOD.
THEME
OUTFITS—
NOT SO GOOD.

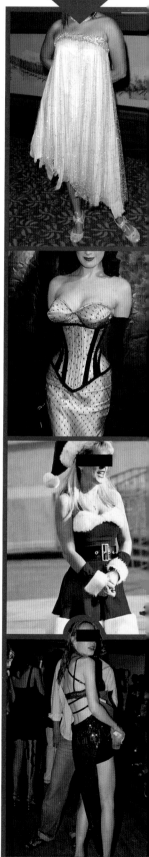

THE BIG DON'TS OF OVER-THE-TOP DRESSING

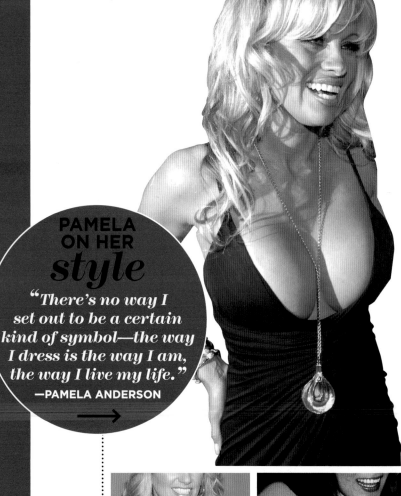

PAMELA ON HER *style*

"There's no way I set out to be a certain kind of symbol—the way I dress is the way I am, the way I live my life."
—PAMELA ANDERSON →

FIRST THERE WAS PAM ANDERSON AND HER SO-DON'T-SHE'S-A-DO STYLE. AND THEN THERE WERE HER CLONES!

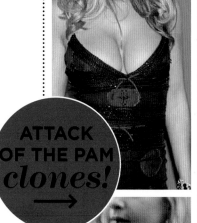

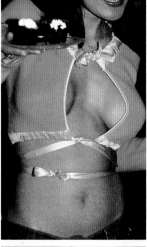

ATTACK OF THE PAM *clones!* →

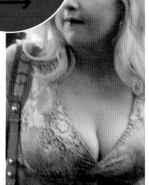

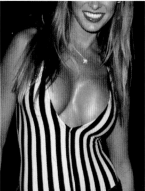

HER
EXTREMELY
SMALL DRESSES

HER
ARABIAN NIGHTS
LOOK

HER TRADEMARK
TIED SHIRT

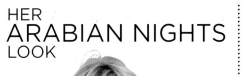

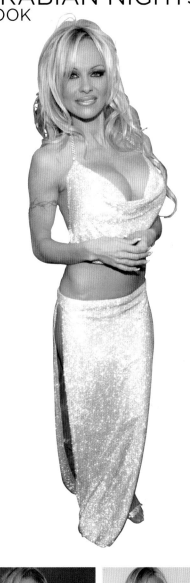

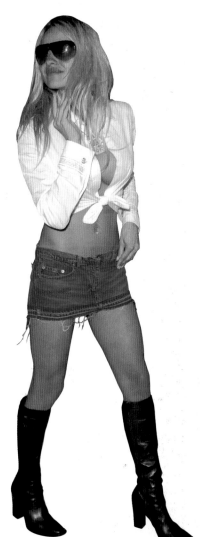

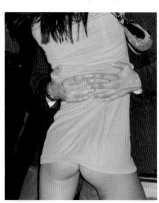

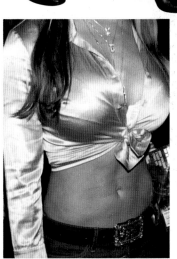

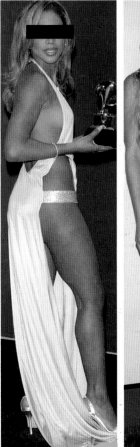

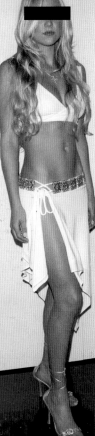

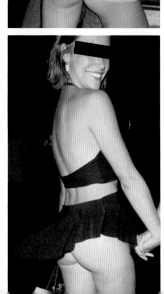

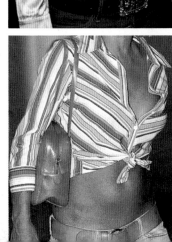

SHOES

THREE CHIC 'N' SEXY NIGHTLIFE SHOES

Sexy footwear doesn't just change the vibe of your outfit—it changes *your* vibe, too, from sexy predator (in stilettos) to ladylike (kitten heels) to rocker girl (cowboy boots, please!). Remember to pretest any shoe at home for comfort, especially strappy sandals. What's the point of fabulous shoes if you can't dance in them?

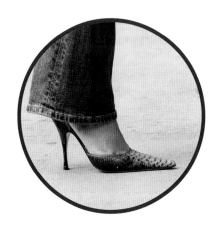

❶

HEELS

- Look for a heel between two and three inches—it'll give you height, comfortably.
- Try a pair in a bright color or pattern that'll take jeans from day to night.
- Invest in a classic black, closed-toe heel in a sexy, non-workday shape, to go with anything.

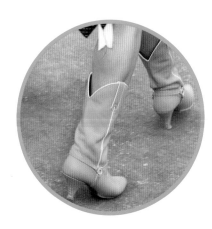

❷

BOOTS

- The heel on dressier boots shouldn't be too chunky. If you like something thicker, make sure it's curvy, like the one at left.
- Tuck in skinny pants or jeans to show them off.
- Try a pair in a bright color or cool pattern—something more fun than what you'd wear to work.

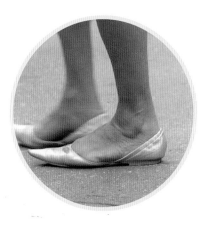

❸

FLATS

- Look for metallic or sparkle-infused flats for nighttime.
- Pointy toes make legs look longer; open sides (called d'Orsay) are sexiest.
- Wear with skirts or slim-cut pants.

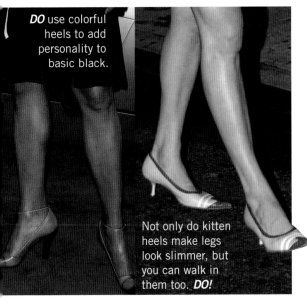

DO use colorful heels to add personality to basic black.

Not only do kitten heels make legs look slimmer, but you can walk in them too. **DO!**

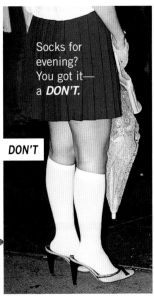

Socks for evening? You got it— a **DON'T.**

DON'T

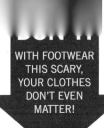

WITH FOOTWEAR THIS SCARY, YOUR CLOTHES DON'T EVEN MATTER!

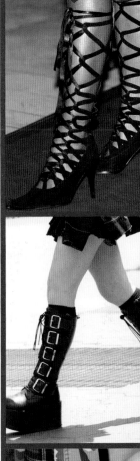

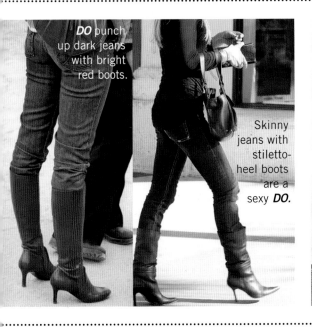

DO punch up dark jeans with bright red boots.

Skinny jeans with stiletto-heel boots are a sexy **DO.**

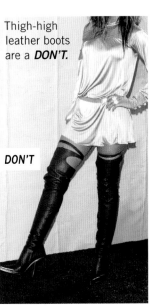

Thigh-high leather boots are a **DON'T.**

DON'T

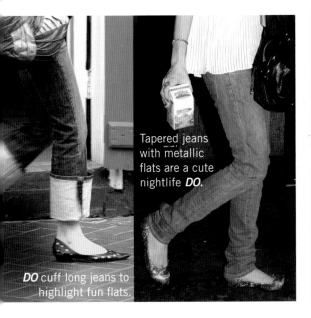

Tapered jeans with metallic flats are a cute nightlife **DO.**

DO cuff long jeans to highlight fun flats.

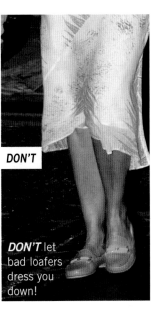

DON'T

DON'T let bad loafers dress you down!

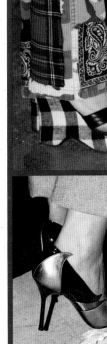

That's toilet paper!

139

ACCENTS

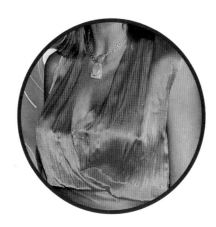

❶ NECKLACES

- Go for versatile styles like dainty gold or silver strands, colorful beads or classic pearls.

- Make sure your necklace complements—but doesn't compete with—what you're wearing.

THREE EVENING ACCESSORIES EVERY WOMAN SHOULD HAVE

Accessories finish and personalize your nighttime look. Add a strong necklace (or several delicate strands) to draw attention to your face. Wear a belt, either low on your hips or cinched at your waist, to highlight your shape. And don't forget a fab little clutch; test-drive a few in the store to find one that holds all of your essentials without looking like an overstuffed burrito.

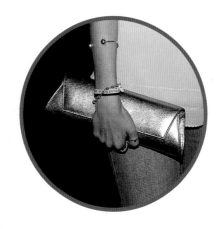

❷ CLUTCHES

- The perfect size will fit all of your necessities, like money, phone, keys and lipstick.

- Try a metallic or embellished clutch for a bit of sparkle.

- Choose a clutch with a wrist strap to keep your hands free.

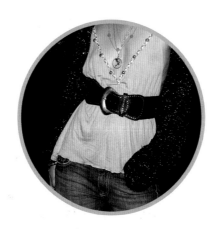

❸ BELTS

- Pick styles and lengths that can be worn at your waist or on your hips.

- Great materials include leather, satin, gold link, *peau de soie* and soft ribbon.

- Try a pretty color or embellished style to add visual interest to a simple outfit.

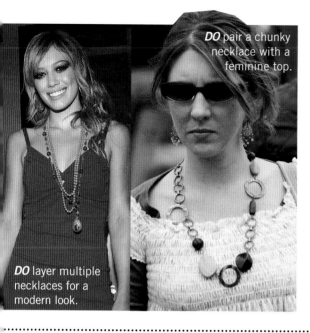

DO pair a chunky necklace with a feminine top.

DO layer multiple necklaces for a modern look.

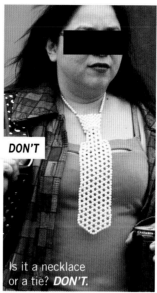

DON'T

Is it a necklace or a tie? DON'T.

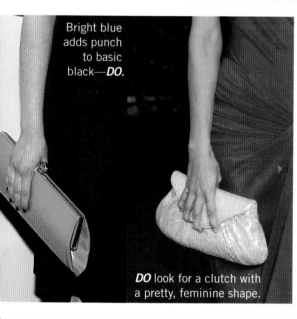

Bright blue adds punch to basic black—DO.

DO look for a clutch with a pretty, feminine shape.

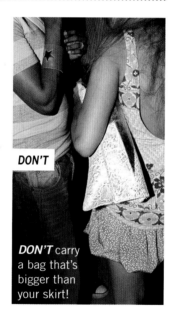

DON'T

DON'T carry a bag that's bigger than your skirt!

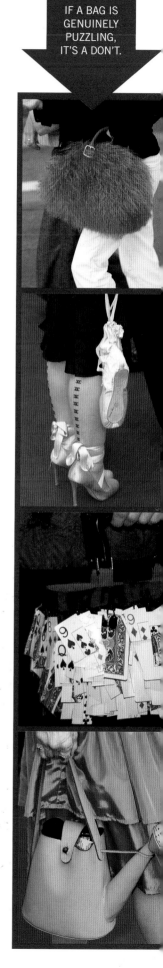

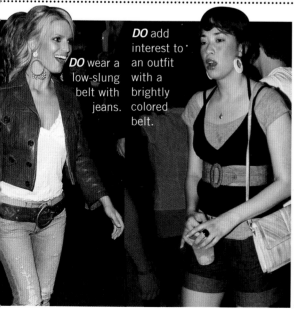

DO wear a low-slung belt with jeans.

DO add interest to an outfit with a brightly colored belt.

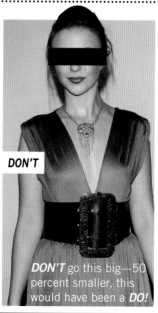

DON'T

DON'T go this big—50 percent smaller, this would have been a DO!

GLAMOUR FACT: JESSICA SIMPSON SAYS THAT SHE TURNS TO VINTAGE PHOTOS OF BRIGITTE BARDOT FOR STYLE INSPIRATION.

YOU'LL BE SEEING YOUR
EX-BOYFRIEND
AT A PARTY

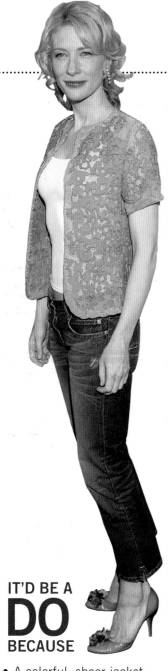

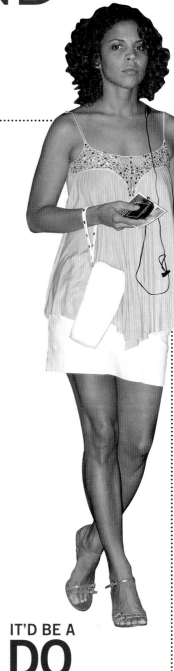

IT'D BE A
DO
BECAUSE

- A printed flippy skirt is sweet and flirty.
- A chunky necklace shows attitude.
- Cowboy boots keep the look casual.

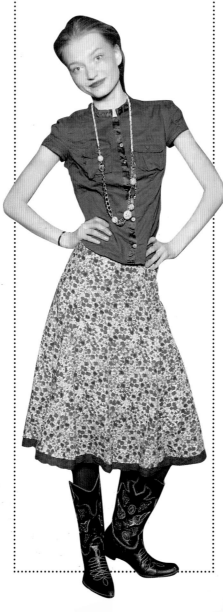

IT'D BE A
DO
BECAUSE

- A colorful, sheer jacket is sexy yet tasteful over a white tank.
- Cropped jeans are perfect for low-key parties.
- Embellished heels are confident and fun.

IT'D BE A
DO
BECAUSE

- This mini is short enough to play up the legs, but long enough to keep it classy.
- Skinny straps show off shoulders.
- A jeweled neckline keeps the focus on top.

YOUR NUMBER-ONE GOAL OF AN EVENING LIKE THIS (BESIDES HAVING FUN): To look Drop. Dead. Gorgeous. But the kind of gorgeous that seems totally effortless, like you just bounded out of bed that way, not the kind that says, "I'm trying really, really hard." THE RULES:
1. No overdressing. Consider the venue; you don't want to show up at a pub crawl in a slinky black dress.
2. Think comfort. After all, you'll never look hot if you're constantly readjusting a strapless bra.
3. Wear something you already know you love—something that makes you feel as beautiful and confident as you are.

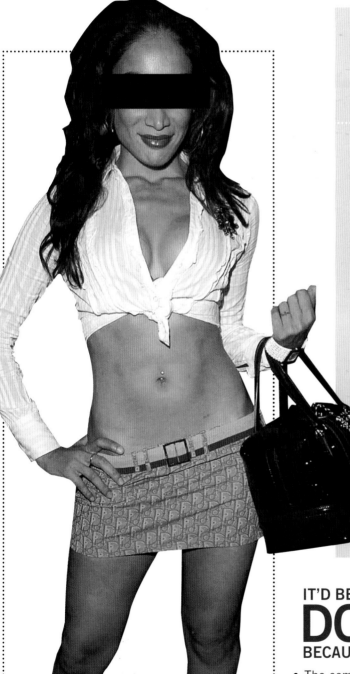

Man-Approved!
FIVE THINGS PRETTY MUCH *ALL* GUYS LIKE TO SEE WOMEN IN

1.
Jeans
Men *understand* jeans and tend to think (rightly or wrongly!) that the women in them are sexy in a low-key, friend way.

2.
White tanks
Survey after *Glamour* survey finds that men like this simple guy-style look. (Don't ask us—maybe they secretly want to date themselves?) Dress it up with a necklace or earrings.

3.
Medium-height heels...
Because too, too high says, "I'm too sexy for you."

4.
...or Chuck Taylor sneaks
Guys wear them—*and* love them on us. Perfect for pool-playing nights.

5.
Cleavage
Not scary over-the-top cleavage, mind you—but *some* cleavage. A-cup, D-cup—it doesn't seem to matter. Guys love it all on you. (Just not your dad.)

IT'D BE A
DON'T
BECAUSE

- The combo of low-cut top, bare midriff and hipster micromini puts way too much skin on display.
- Face it: If this is what would get your ex's attention, you're lucky he's an "ex."

YOU'RE INVITED TO A
POSH COCKTAIL PARTY

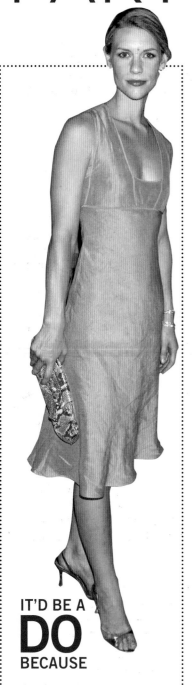

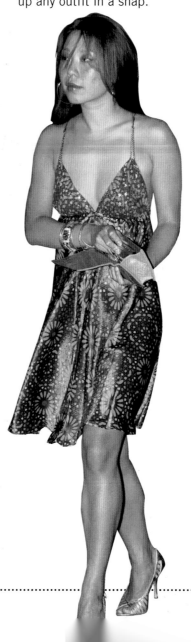

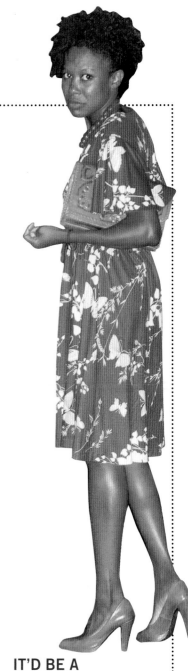

IT'D BE A
DO
BECAUSE

- It's low-cut but covers front and sides.
- Flowy, patterned fabric is flirty.
- Simple gold heels dress up any outfit in a snap.

IT'D BE A
DO
BECAUSE

- A bright look stands out in a sea of black.
- Pointed-toe slingbacks elongate legs.
- An embellished clutch instantly signals "fancy."

IT'D BE A
DO
BECAUSE

- The vintage dress shows off personal style.
- The classic heels keep focus on that show-piece dress!

A COCKTAIL PARTY IS ONE GREAT EXCUSE TO GET ALL-OUT DRESSY—YOU DON'T WANT to step out the door in the same clothes you'd wear for casual drinks with friends. Instead, follow these rules to amp up your look: 1. Even if you just pair flashy heels with jeans, elevate your standard night uniform with a definitively dressy touch. 2. Go for glam jewelry and bags that you'd *never* wear to work—you'll instantly feel special. 3. Choose your footwear wisely. Chances are you'll be standing all evening, so make sure you're in *comfortable* heels.

IT'D BE A
DON'T
BECAUSE

- The dress is too short and the cap's too sporty if she were going to a cocktail party.
- Metallic dress + metallic tights + metallic bag = metallic overload.

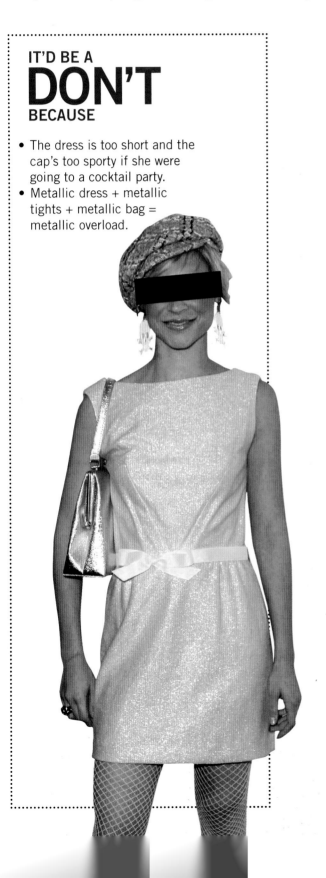

Last All Night
FOUR TRICKS TO STAY PARTY-FRESH TILL THE WEE HOURS

1.
Don't mix drinks
Stick with one type, and have a glass of water between cocktails.

2.
Manage your heels
Carry clear Band-Aids if this is a pair's first public outing, and try sticking in little pads to give the balls of your feet some cushioning.

3.
Scent yourself
Carry an atomizer of your favorite fragrance for a quick pick-me-up.

4.
Eat!
Even (especially!) if all they're serving is pigs in a blanket, make sure you're not drinking on an empty stomach.

Bling 101
THREE PIECES OF JEWELRY THAT CAN MAKE YOUR WHOLE LOOK

1.
Multiple necklaces
Three or four chains of various lengths dress up your neck and shoulders.

2.
Chandelier earrings
Large, dangling ones catch the light and frame your face.

3.
A statement bracelet
A chunky one or several small bands highlight pretty, bare arms.

IS IT A DO OR A DON'T?

LEATHER PANTS

A sleek pair of leather pants can be a great nightlife investment. Buy the best-quality leather you can afford—in go-with-everything black or deep brown. Wear them with a fitted tee and heels to keep them edgy, or with a floaty top for a more feminine look.

OUR VERDICT:
mostly a DO

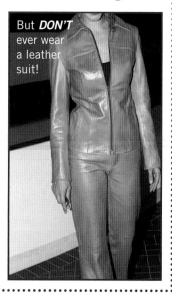

But **DON'T** ever wear a leather suit!

DO pair skinny black leather pants and a rocker T-shirt.

LEGGINGS

Worn the right way, leggings are now a DO: They look great under a skirt or dress, especially if you're shy about showing your legs. Or try them under a long tunic top with a belt. Finish with flats and you're good to go. But DON'T try to wear them with a short top—and avoid leggings like the see-through ones at right.

OUR VERDICT:
often a DON'T

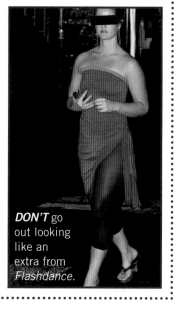

DON'T go out looking like an extra from *Flashdance.*

DO wear a flowy dress over black capri leggings.

SUNGLASSES AT NIGHT

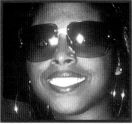
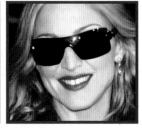
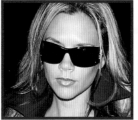
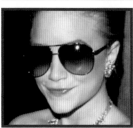
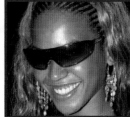
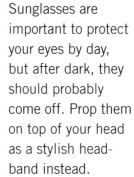
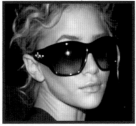

Sunglasses are important to protect your eyes by day, but after dark, they should probably come off. Prop them on top of your head as a stylish head-band instead.

OUR VERDICT:
a DO, but impractical

DRESS OVER PANTS

A dress worn over pants is chic and modern for night if you keep the proportions in balance. Go for an above-the-knee-length dress, and pair it with heels and skinny jeans or pants. Avoid either voluminous dresses or wide pants or you'll be drowning in fabric.

OUR VERDICT:
a DO

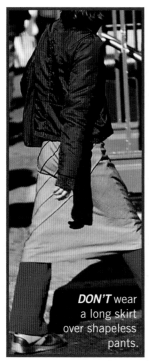

DON'T wear a long skirt over shapeless pants.

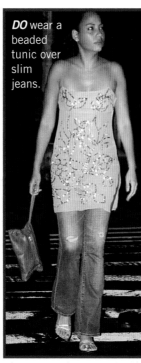

DO wear a beaded tunic over slim jeans.

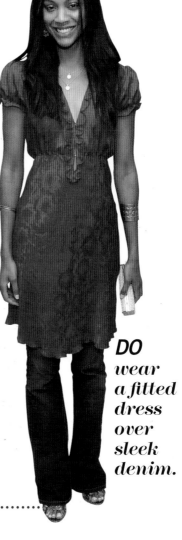

DO *wear a fitted dress over sleek denim.*

ALWAYS A DO AT NIGHT

A killer pair of heels

The perfect Little Black Dress

A pair of jeans that hug you in all the right places

One great piece of "statement" jewelry

Bolder-than-day makeup that puts the focus on either your lips or eyes

A top that showcases your best asset: neck, back, shoulders or arms

"I WANT TO LOOK VINTAGE-CHIC!"

Of her dowdy "before" outfit, below, Sarah says, "I was going for vintage but wound up looking old-fashioned." Although she loves being 5'9", finding pants long enough is tough, she says: "I always wind up wearing skirts and dresses." So she needs fun, feminine pieces that look *modern*. Done!

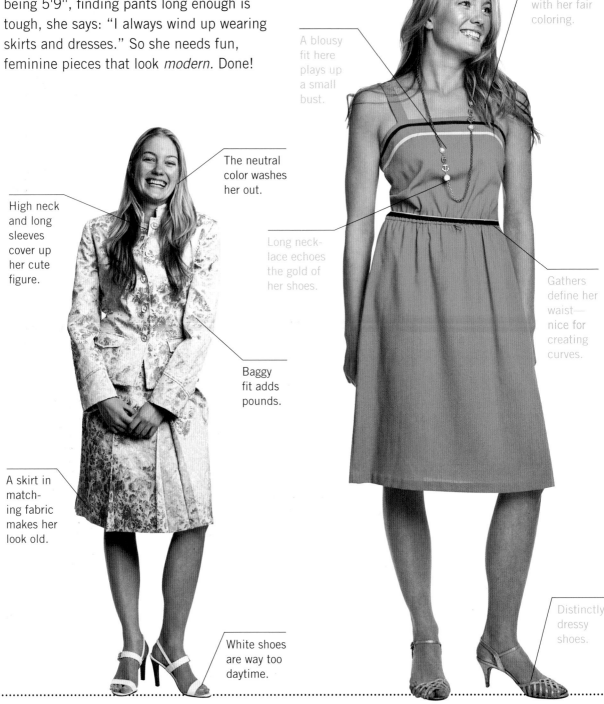

The green looks great with her fair coloring.

A blousy fit here plays up a small bust.

The neutral color washes her out.

High neck and long sleeves cover up her cute figure.

Long neck-lace echoes the gold of her shoes.

Baggy fit adds pounds.

A skirt in matching fabric makes her look old.

Gathers define her waist— nice for creating curves.

White shoes are way too daytime.

Distinctly dressy shoes.

BEFORE:
Sarah Robinson, 26

CASUAL DINNER

"I love this dress because it is so bright and comfortable yet still looks tailored."

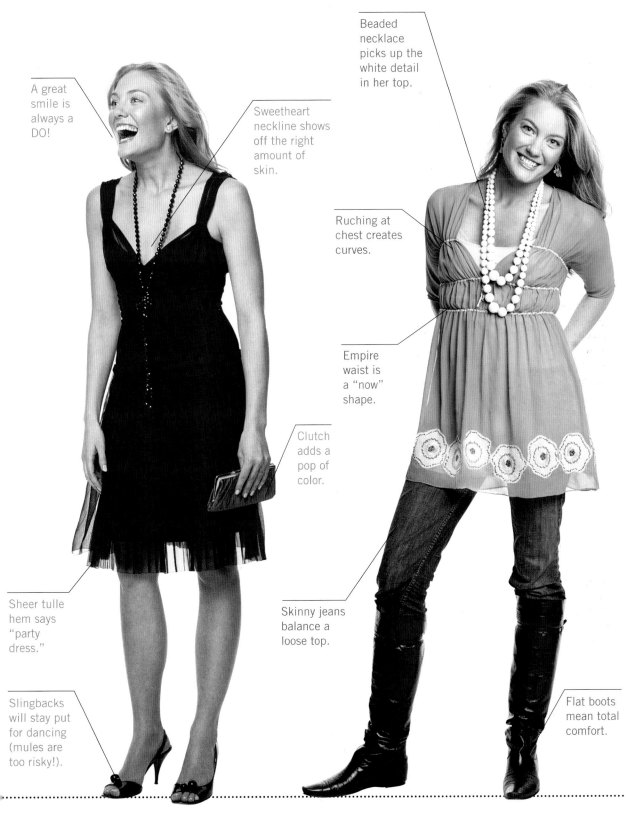

A great smile is always a DO!

Sweetheart neckline shows off the right amount of skin.

Clutch adds a pop of color.

Sheer tulle hem says "party dress."

Slingbacks will stay put for dancing (mules are too risky!).

Beaded necklace picks up the white detail in her top.

Ruching at chest creates curves.

Empire waist is a "now" shape.

Skinny jeans balance a loose top.

Flat boots mean total comfort.

COCKTAILS

"It's perfect for a friend's birthday party!"

MOVIE WITH FRIENDS

"The embroidery around the bottom adds a vintage feel that's casual enough for a movie but fancy enough if we go out after."

"NO MORE FIGHTING MY CURVES!"

This Connecticut innkeeper's closet was packed with clothes that didn't flatter her voluptuous figure. Of her shirt, below, she says, "I bought it because it disguised my stomach but still showed my cleavage." True, but any positive effects are canceled out by the unflattering satiny fabric and bustline gathering. Kathryn's new clothes are a lot more curve-friendly—better fitting and dramatically enhancing.

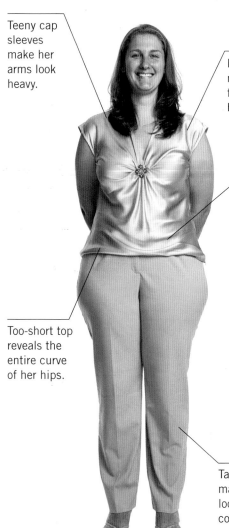

Teeny cap sleeves make her arms look heavy.

Pale color makes her fade into the background.

Halter top + large bust = great fit!

Black makes her creamy skin stand out.

Longer shirt covers the midsection.

Shiny material can add inches, plus this clings in all the wrong places.

Too-short top reveals the entire curve of her hips.

Boot-cut jeans balance out her proportions.

Tapered legs make her hips look wider by comparison.

BEFORE:
Kathryn Brewster, 24

BARHOPPING WITH FRIENDS
"This outfit is so easy to put together and it looks absolutely great. Plus, the dark jeans make my legs look long and lean."

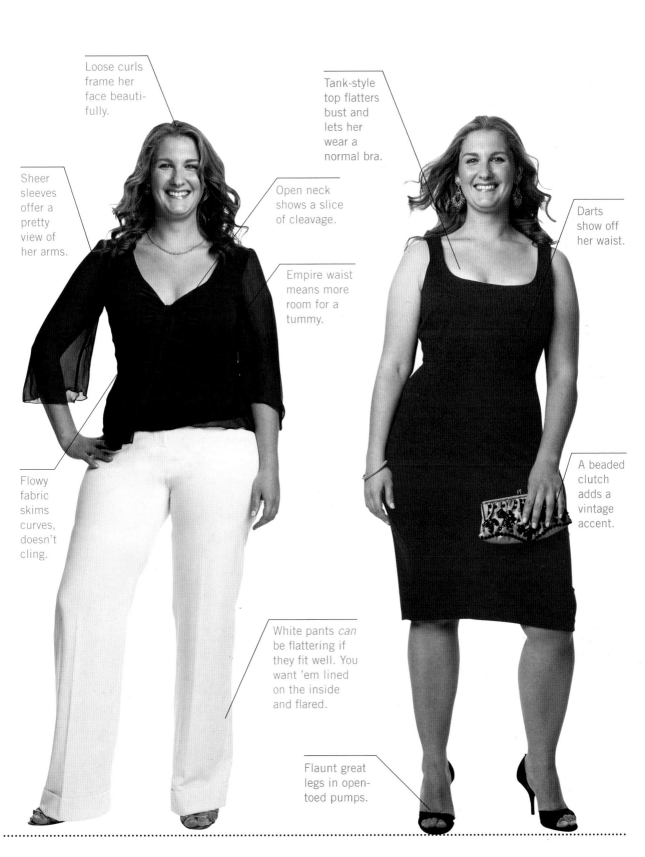

Loose curls frame her face beautifully.

Sheer sleeves offer a pretty view of her arms.

Flowy fabric skims curves, doesn't cling.

Open neck shows a slice of cleavage.

Empire waist means more room for a tummy.

White pants *can* be flattering if they fit well. You want 'em lined on the inside and flared.

Tank-style top flatters bust and lets her wear a normal bra.

Darts show off her waist.

A beaded clutch adds a vintage accent.

Flaunt great legs in open-toed pumps.

DINNER DATE

"Very comfortable—the pants are fitted and accentuate my shape in a good way."

COCKTAIL PARTY

"I'm full-figured, and I'm not trying to hide that. This is sexy and hugs my curves."

151

"MAKE ME ELEGANT!"

Since Stephanie handles celebrity and VIP accounts for a designer clothing brand, a lot of her nighttime activities involve entertaining clients. She knows the short-waisted top and low-rise jeans combo below is a definite DON'T, especially because it makes her petite, curvy figure look pudgy, and she's ready to upgrade her look. "I can't stand when chub hangs off the sides of jeans!" Stephanie says. Here, she's in evening outfits that are chic enough for her fanciest clients, yet still comfortable.

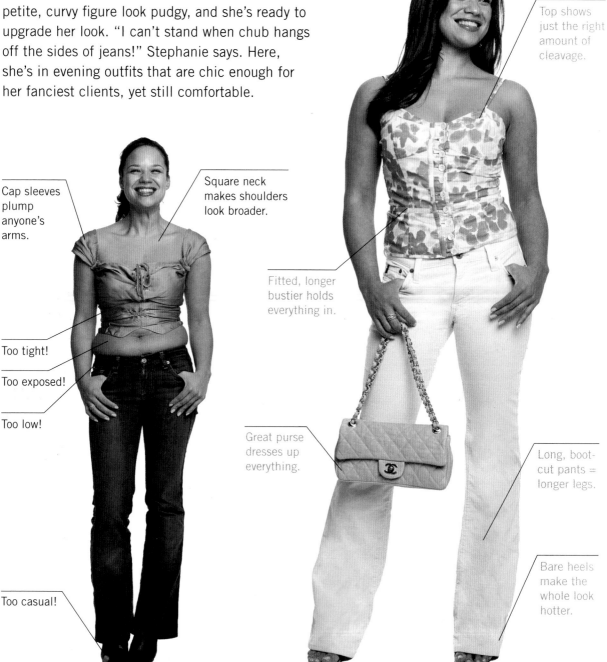

Long, shiny hair is a can't-miss accessory.

Top shows just the right amount of cleavage.

Cap sleeves plump anyone's arms.

Square neck makes shoulders look broader.

Fitted, longer bustier holds everything in.

Too tight!

Too exposed!

Too low!

Great purse dresses up everything.

Long, boot-cut pants = longer legs.

Too casual!

Bare heels make the whole look hotter.

BEFORE:
Stephanie Anson, 26

ROOFTOP DRINKS

"I love form-fitting bustier tops paired with skinny pants—I'm only 5'1", and this outfit elongates my body."

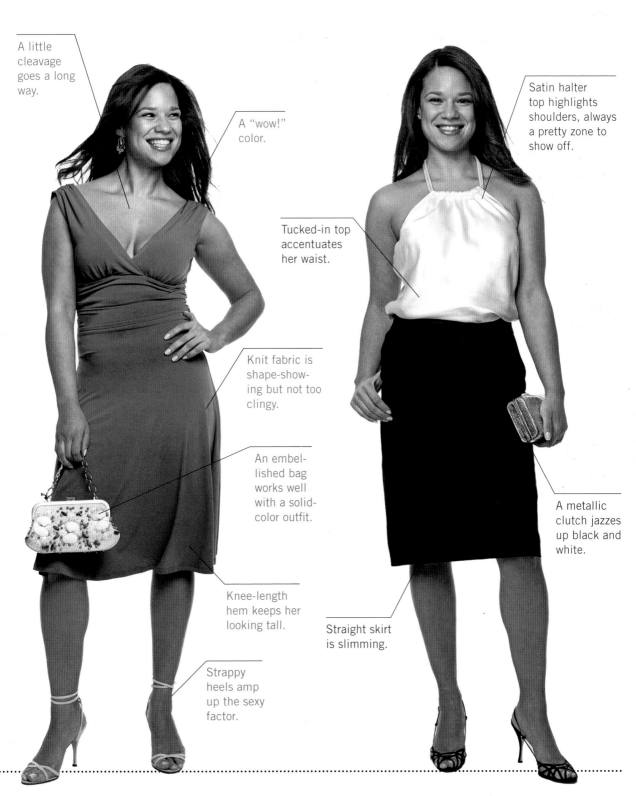

A little cleavage goes a long way.

A "wow!" color.

Satin halter top highlights shoulders, always a pretty zone to show off.

Tucked-in top accentuates her waist.

Knit fabric is shape-show-ing but not too clingy.

An embel-lished bag works well with a solid-color outfit.

A metallic clutch jazzes up black and white.

Knee-length hem keeps her looking tall.

Straight skirt is slimming.

Strappy heels amp up the sexy factor.

FRIDAY AFTER WORK

"This is a flirty, girly outfit that makes me feel sexy. Plus, the color is bold and eye-catching."

DRINKS WITH VIPs

"This isn't too showy or loud, but under-stated, simple and non-revealing."

HALL OF shame

DOUBLE DON'TS!
WHAT HAPPENS WHEN GOOD COUPLES WEAR BAD THINGS?

DON'T imagine what's lurking in all those dread-locks—ewww.

Too many flowers. Sorry—it's a **DON'T**.

Is it Halloween? No? Then **DON'T!**

DON'T flaunt your pumped-up pecs—Too Much Information!

Unless you two are an official rodeo act, **DON'T.**

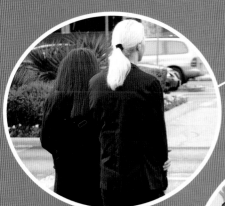

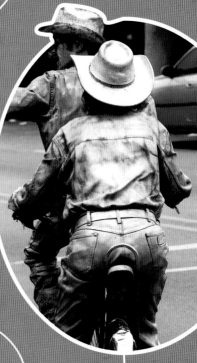

We're pretty sure these hair colors **DON'T** occur in nature.

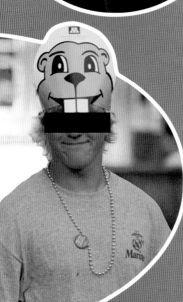

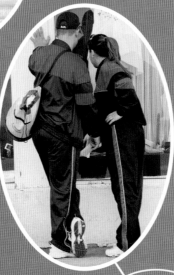

It's fine to work out together, just **DON'T** do it in his-and-hers tracksuits.

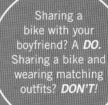

Sharing a bike with your boyfriend? A **DO.** Sharing a bike and wearing matching outfits? **DON'T!**

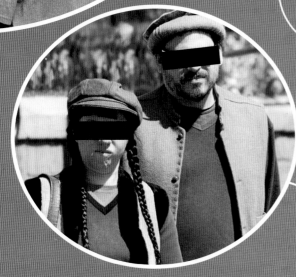

DON'T pair up in blah brown caps and tops.

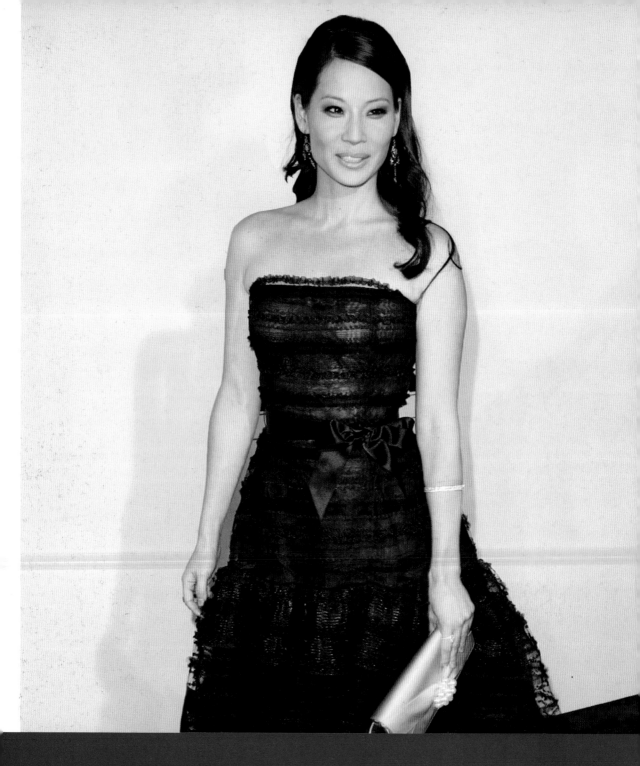

YOUR

DO

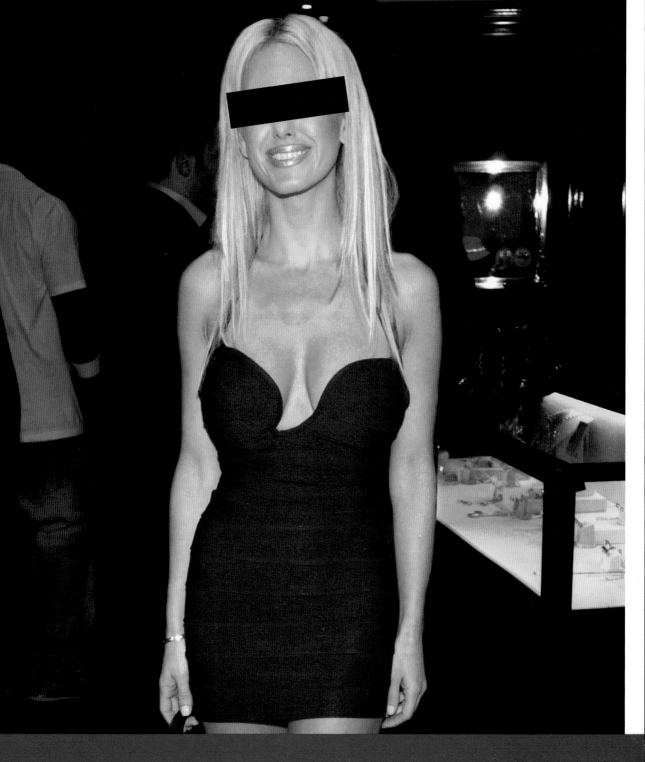

SPECIAL EVENTS

WHAT TO WEAR FOR LIFE'S TRICKIEST OCCASIONS

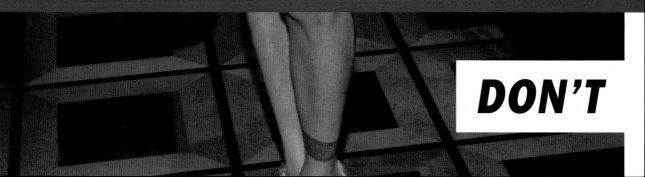

DON'T

THE RULES

*for special events, weddings,
reunions and big-deal parties*

WHEN IN DOUBT, DRESS UP.

*Being a little too fancy is always better
than being the only one in jeans.*

OWN ONE AMAZING COCKTAIL DRESS.

*It should make you look and feel like
you could conquer the universe (or at least the room).*

MIX POSH AND CASUAL STUFF.

*It's a way to dress up without feeling old-school formal.
Try a plain turtleneck with your ball skirt (as opposed to an
equally dressy top), or simple black pants with a sequined top.*

THINK LONG-TERM WITH
SPECIAL-EVENT PURCHASES.

*Big-night clothes are pricey, yes, but consider
them investments in your social life (bonus: no broker fees!).
Go for classic shapes in neutral colors so that you can make
them look new with each accessory change.*

STOCK UP ON PRETTY WRAPS.

*A flash of color in cashmere, wool or silk will score you style
points and shield you from nippy rooms and night air.*

STEP UP YOUR JEWELRY . . .

*Now's the time to take out the quality pieces that you
have socked away, like pearl or diamond studs, gold bangles,
a platinum watch from your grandmother. If you're into
splashy costume stuff, limit it to one statement-making piece.*

. . . AND YOUR COAT.

*Sure, the high-low mix of a parka and a slinky dress
looks great on runway models, but for the rest of us, a belted
black trench is the perfect dressy topper.*

DON'T BUY ANYTHING YOU NEED
TO LOSE WEIGHT TO FIT INTO.

*You tell yourself you'll diet your way into it, but why?
The last thing you want is to reach the big day and discover
you need pliers to zip up your dream dress. Buy what fits.*

 IF YOU CAN FOLLOW ONLY ONE RULE, THIS IS IT!

REMEMBER, LINGERIE COUNTS.

*Nighttime clothes often pose a set of lingerie challenges totally
different from your day stuff—you might need a halter or
something strapless on top; a bulge-control or entirely
seamless piece on the bottom. The point: Shop for these pieces
in advance, and wear them when you try on big-night outfits.*

GO FOR LOOK-AT-ME SHOES.

*Use them to play off your clothes: Try a patterned fabric
with a solid dress, a brilliant color with a black outfit or
a jewel-encrusted pair with a classic pantsuit.*

SKIRTS

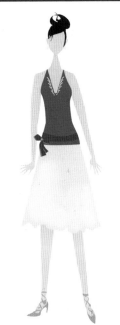

1 SATIN SKIRT

- Choose knee-length—always in style.
- Wear it with a fitted top for maximum flattery.
- Avoid extremely tight, tapered pencil-skirt shapes—the shiny fabric will only enlarge curves.

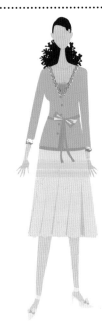

2 CIRCLE SKIRT

- Go for full shapes that hit midshin.
- Find one that is fitted through the hips.
- Balance the skirt's fullness with a snug top.

THREE DRESSY SKIRTS

A closet staple, skirts can be gussied up for black-tie affairs or dressed down for more casual "special events" (say, a reunion dinner). The smartest kind to own: a satin skirt (more versatile than you think), a circle skirt (in silk or satin) and a ball skirt (to head off black-tie panic for the rest of your life).

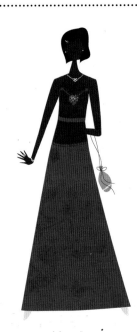

3 BALL SKIRT

- Get one with a fitted, higher waist.
- Pair with a clingy shirt, a simple blouse or even a turtleneck. (Remember Sharon Stone at the Oscars with her full skirt and Gap turtleneck?)
- Find one that doesn't quite skim the floor so your shoes peek out.

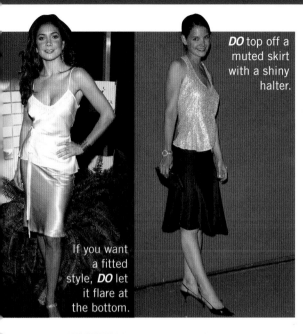

DO top off a muted skirt with a shiny halter.

If you want a fitted style, *DO* let it flare at the bottom.

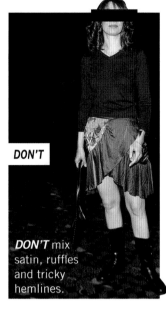

DON'T

DON'T mix satin, ruffles and tricky hemlines.

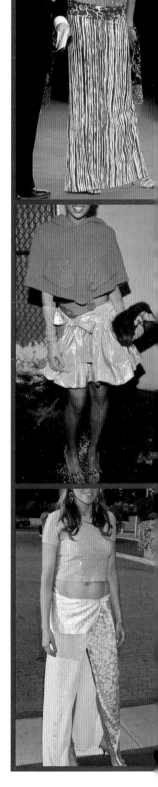

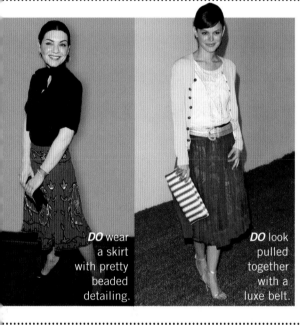

DO wear a skirt with pretty beaded detailing.

DO look pulled together with a luxe belt.

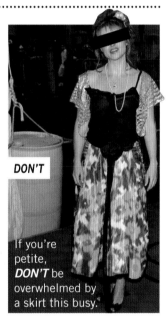

DON'T

If you're petite, *DON'T* be overwhelmed by a skirt this busy.

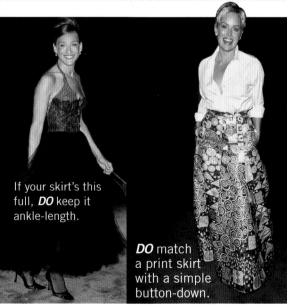

If your skirt's this full, *DO* keep it ankle-length.

DO match a print skirt with a simple button-down.

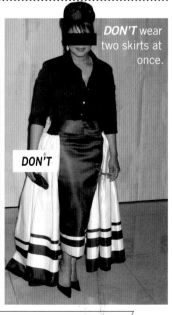

DON'T wear two skirts at once.

DON'T

DRESSES

THREE SPECIAL DRESSES WORTH OWNING

They'll save your butt (and flatter it), so plan to invest in a trip to the tailor to perfect the fit. Worth knowing: While he or she can change skirt length, strap length and basic waist shape without much ado, there are some things that cannot be fixed, like too-big armholes or fabric that pulls across your legs or tummy. And always sit in the dress to make sure the waist and torso are comfortable.

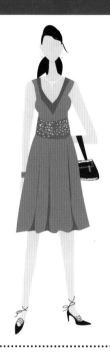

1 COCKTAIL

- Look for a classic style in a fabric that's fancier than your work dresses.
- Choose one with subtle embellishments—less is more if you want to wear this baby more than once.
- To dress up, pair with colored shoes or glitzy jewelry.

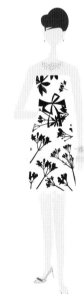

2 STRAPLESS

- Make sure that it's tight enough across the chest to stay put when you wave.
- Go for one with boning for extra support—and invest in a stay-put strapless bra!
- Check your rear view; strapless dresses can give you back cleavage if they're too tight. Yikes!

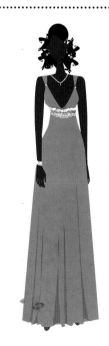

3 GOWN

- Find a body-conscious cut in a fluid material.
- Try out an interesting neckline that shows off skin—it will keep you from looking too covered-up.
- Finish with great accessories: a small bag, delicate jewelry and pretty shoes.

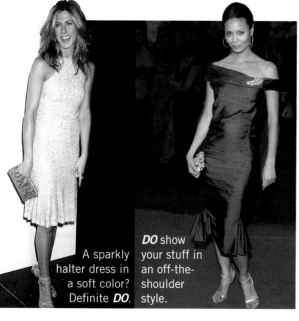

A sparkly halter dress in a soft color? Definite **DO**.

DO show your stuff in an off-the-shoulder style.

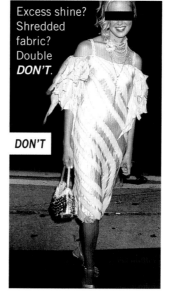

Excess shine? Shredded fabric? Double **DON'T**.

DON'T

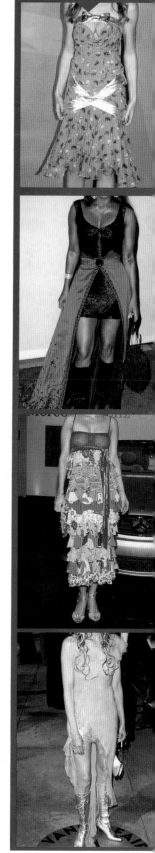

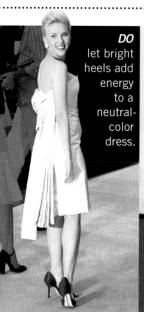

DO let bright heels add energy to a neutral-color dress.

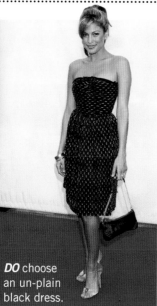

DO choose an un-plain black dress.

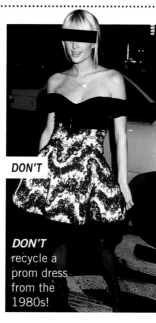

DON'T

DON'T recycle a prom dress from the 1980s!

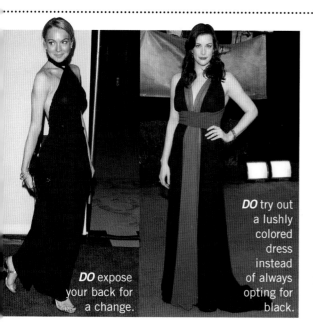

DO expose your back for a change.

DO try out a lushly colored dress instead of always opting for black.

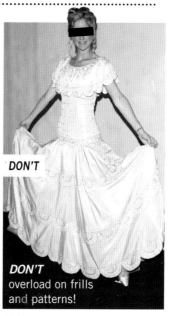

DON'T

DON'T overload on frills and patterns!

PANTS

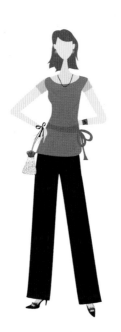

❶

TROUSER

- The point here is a sleek, flat-front fit.

- Select classic, elegant fabrics like wool crepe, silk and satin.

- Pair with an un-plain top and elegant shoes.

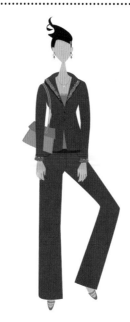

❷

PANTSUIT

- Make sure the pants are slim and form-hugging.

- Choose a jacket that's fitted and has one or two buttons— it'll look sexier.

- Wear it with high heels to keep from looking too menswear-y.

- No tweed, no cotton!

THREE
FORMAL PANTS

They can be just as dressy as gowns—assuming that you ditch the canvas, cotton and cargo styles in favor of special fabrics like velvet, matte silk or fine wool. Pair with sparkly shirts, luxurious jackets and gorgeous shoes.

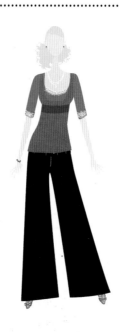

❸

WIDE-LEG

- Pick fabrics that drape— stiff, wide legs are tricky.

- Combine with a fitted top for a tailored, not schlumpy, look.

- Choose a top that's somewhat bare—it'll balance the full leg.

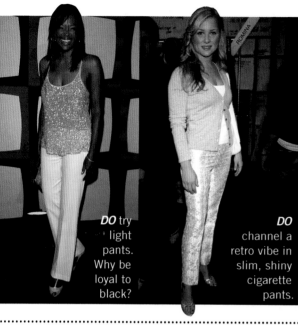

DO try light pants. Why be loyal to black?

DO channel a retro vibe in slim, shiny cigarette pants.

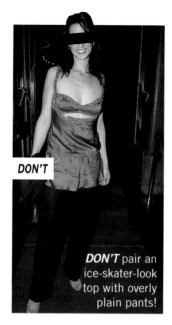

DON'T

DON'T pair an ice-skater-look top with overly plain pants!

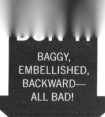

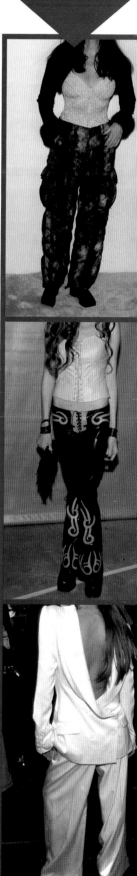

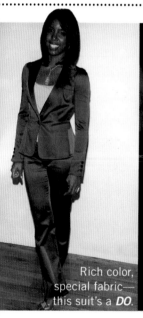

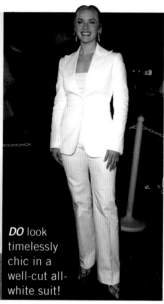

Rich color, special fabric— this suit's a **DO**.

DO look timelessly chic in a well-cut all-white suit!

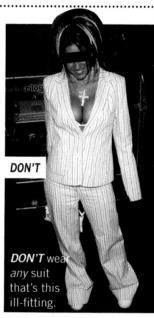

DON'T

DON'T wear *any* suit that's this ill-fitting.

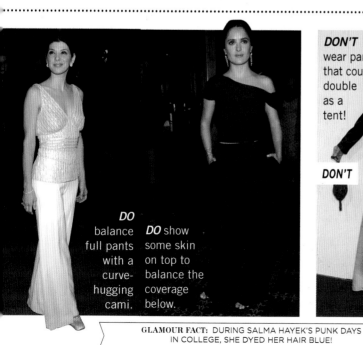

DO balance full pants with a curve-hugging cami.

DO show some skin on top to balance the coverage below.

DON'T wear pants that could double as a tent!

DON'T

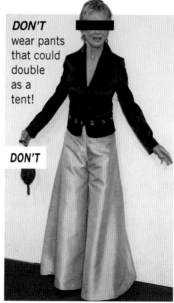

GLAMOUR FACT: DURING SALMA HAYEK'S PUNK DAYS IN COLLEGE, SHE DYED HER HAIR BLUE!

SHOES

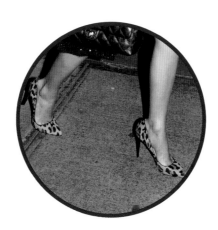

❶ PUMPS

- Best comfort test: Get off the cushy carpet and walk around on the hard floor before you buy.
- Choose a style with a little "toe cleavage"—it slims your ankles and looks sexy!
- Pair with longer skirts, dresses and pants—no minis.

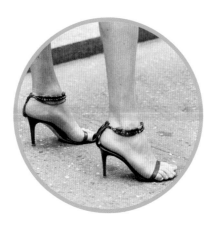

❷ STRAPPY SANDALS

- Show your elegance with thin straps and narrow heels.
- Beware that ankle straps can make your legs appear shorter.
- Don't forget a pedicure! (It makes even cheap shoes look pricey.)

THREE
SEXY SHOES

You know you love heels, and why wouldn't you? They can glam up any outfit, take you from staid to sexy and set you apart from the crowd—all in as long as it takes to slip 'em on. Only caveat: You *must* be able to walk in them without hanging on to a wall (or a man).

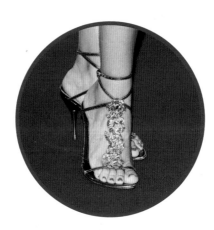

❸ EMBELLISHED

- Go for special details that aren't garish and won't overwhelm your outfit.
- Opt for strappy heels, flats or pumps.
- Jazz up a simple dress with the same.

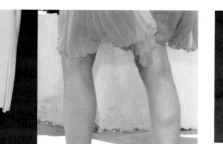

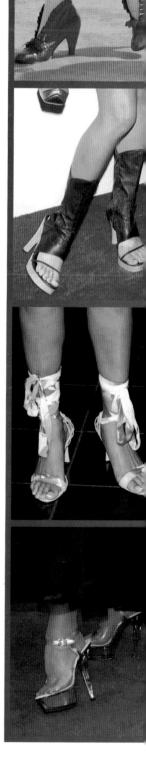

A streamlined black pump is always a **DO**.

If you're going to match your skirt and shoe, **DO** make sure they're the exact same color.

DON'T

DON'T wear Wicked Witch of the West shoes!

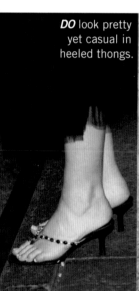

DO look pretty yet casual in heeled thongs.

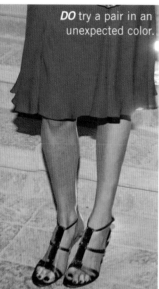

DO try a pair in an unexpected color.

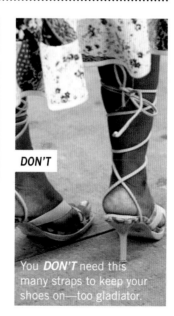

DON'T

You **DON'T** need this many straps to keep your shoes on—too gladiator.

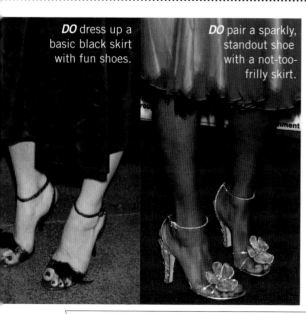

DO dress up a basic black skirt with fun shoes.

DO pair a sparkly, standout shoe with a not-too-frilly skirt.

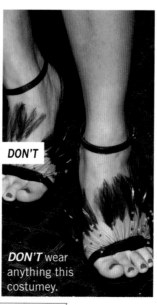

DON'T

DON'T wear anything this costumey.

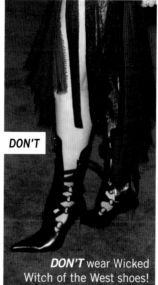

GLAMOUR FACT: IN THE 1960s, THE AVERAGE SHOE SIZE FOR AN ADULT WOMAN WAS 5½; IN 2004, IT WAS 8½.

HAIR

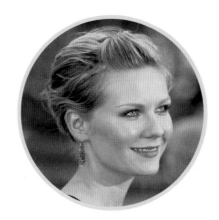

1
UPDO

- Try a loose, not-so-perfect bun for a more modern look.
- Avoid excessive hairspray or pinning—no need to look stiff!
- An updo's a sophisticated option for longer hair.

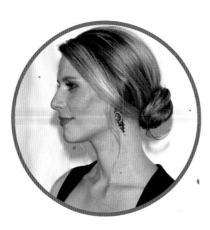

2
CHIGNON

- Draw attention to your neck with a sleek, low twist.
- Add sparkle with a metallic or beaded hair clip.
- To make it even prettier, leave out a few tendrils.

THREE BIG-NIGHT STYLES

Luckily, overly shellacked, can't-touch-your-hair, high-maintenance styles have gone the way of the scrunchie. These days, the easiest, most classic looks get the biggest raves. One simple tweak: Pulled-back hair highlights your face, back, neck, earrings—*everything.*

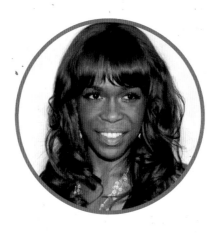

3
LONG CURLS

- Channel classic Hollywood glamour with loose, romantic curls.
- Get soft layers to frame your face.
- Boost shine and hold with mousse or pomade.

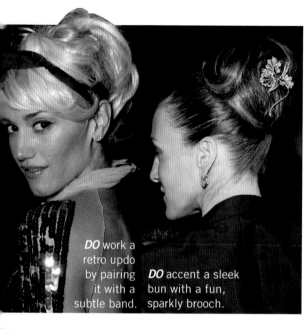

DO work a retro updo by pairing it with a subtle band.

DO accent a sleek bun with a fun, sparkly brooch.

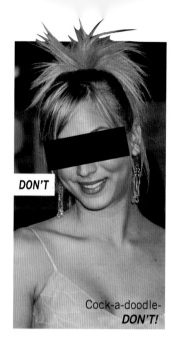

DON'T

Cock-a-doodle-**DON'T!**

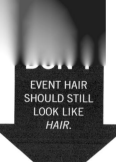

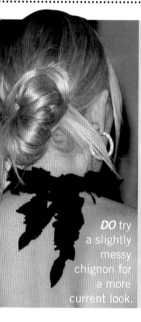

DO try a slightly messy chignon for a more current look.

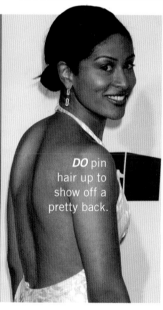

DO pin hair up to show off a pretty back.

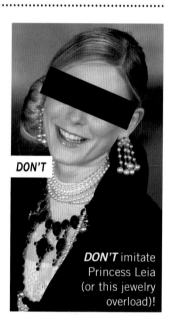

DON'T

DON'T imitate Princess Leia (or this jewelry overload)!

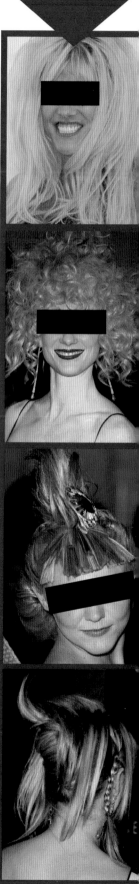

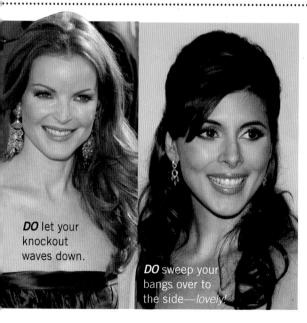

DO let your knockout waves down.

DO sweep your bangs over to the side—*lovely!*

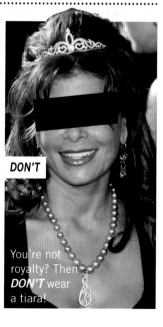

DON'T

You're not royalty? Then **DON'T** wear a tiara!

IT'S YOUR HIGH-SCHOOL
REUNION

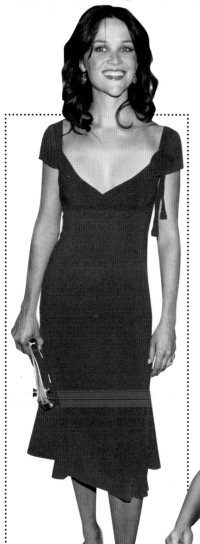

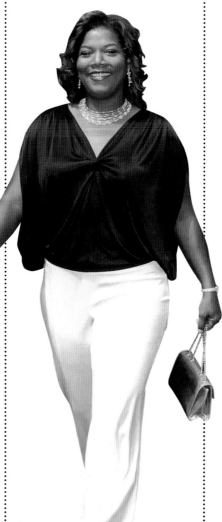

IT'D BE A
DO
BECAUSE

- Sleek, perfect-fit pants are chic.
- A flowy, un-plain blouse provides great balance.
- The gold bag and jewelry dress up her look.

IT'D BE A
DO
BECAUSE

- A bold color signals confidence.
- A slim cut emphasizes your curves. (You've improved since high school—show it!)
- Her hair's casual—that keeps the look from being *too* formal.

IT'D BE A
DO
BECAUSE

- The muted color combo is sophisticated.
- A feminine skirt is fresh-looking, not uptight.
- The simple top makes her outfit not-formal.
- A cute clutch holds all the essentials.

THIS IS ONE OF THE WORLD'S TRICKIEST FASHION MOMENTS, and what's appropriate can range from jeans (for a daytime, outdoor thing) to a cocktail dress (for the more typical Saturday-night soirée). Good rules for wherever you're going: 1. Aim for a look that's up-to-date, but not excessively trendy. 2. Don't overdress. (A too-formal ensemble screams, "I've been worrying about this night for years!") 3. Be just sexy *enough*. Didn't we all learn in high school that flashing lots of skin won't get us the guys who are *really* worth getting?

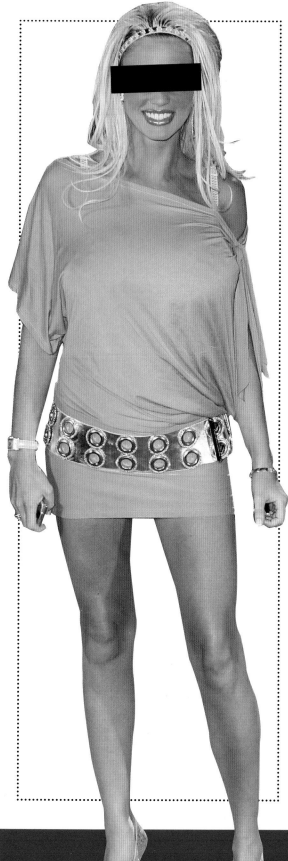

Time Warp!
FIVE TRENDS YOU DON'T WANT TO RESURRECT

1.
Overstyled hair
A super-permed or bleached 'do should be traded in for a great cut and a good blow-out.

2.
Clunky shoes
They may have made a statement in 1992, but your best bet now is a killer pair of sexy heels.

3.
Too much jewelry
Lose the stackable bangles, huge earrings and major rings in favor of something more delicate.

4.
Eye makeup overload
Steer clear of crazy mascara and layers of shadow: Highlight your eyes, don't traumatize them!

5.
XXL outfits
Who cares if you don't have a 16-year-old's body? You don't have her insecurities, either. So no need to cover up your supposed "flaws" with baggy, saggy clothes.

IT'D BE A
DON'T
BECAUSE

- She's in serious danger of flashing fellow dancers—not the desired effect if she were reunion-bound.
- The belt is too Wonder Woman— and a sparkly headband? Even if you *were* homecoming queen, leave it at home.

IT'S
NEW YEAR'S EVE

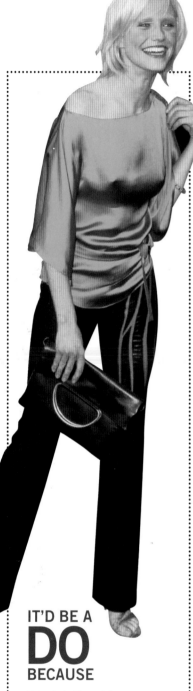

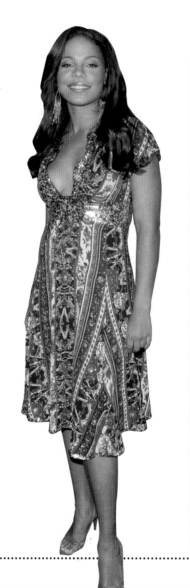

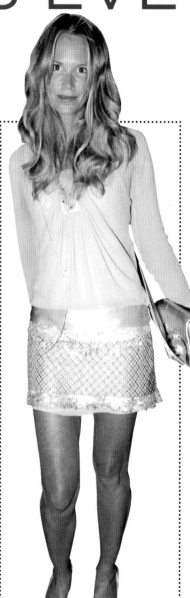

IT'D BE A
DO
BECAUSE

- The low neckline (which shows off a great décolletage) is offset by the longer length.
- It's dressy but not over-the-top.
- The glittery shoes are adorable!

IT'D BE A
DO
BECAUSE

- Black tailored trousers are comfy and sleek.
- A vibrant top is always party-worthy.
- Off the shoulder is sexy but safe.

IT'D BE A
DO
BECAUSE

- New Year's Eve is the perfect time to wear something sparkly.
- Worn with a non-bare top, a mini is fun, not trashy.
- Hair and makeup are natural.

EVERY YEAR, THIS HOLIDAY SERVES AS ONE GLORIFIED EXCUSE TO PARTY—and every year, the what-to-wear worries set in somewhere around Thanksgiving. Advice: Research your party before planning your outfit. What's the dress code? Is there a theme? The night is bound to be long, so make sure you're wearing comfy stuff that's easy to move in and won't show everything when you hit the dance floor after a few too many glasses of whatever. But it *is* a celebration! Get creative and add some sparkle.

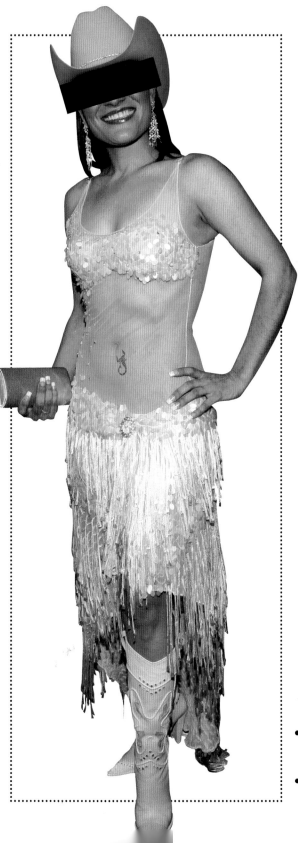

Are You Party-Ready?
FIVE THINGS TO CHECK OUT IN THE MIRROR

1.
Makeup
Evening calls for a bit more color, so try a smoky eye or bold lip. And if you're a shimmer addict, tonight you can wear it with abandon, so dust on décolletage, brow bone or temples.

2.
Shoes
Go wild with color, sparkle and prints, but beware of too-high heels that'll force you to sit down way before the ball drops.

3.
Hair
Pull it back, put it up, wear it down. Just do something that's *not* your everyday style.

4.
Lingerie
You'll feel instantly dressy and celebratory in your sexiest stuff!

5.
Jewelry
Wear one big piece of bling, be it rhinestone drop earrings, a gaggle of gold chains or a sparkly brooch.

IT'D BE A
DON'T
BECAUSE

- Whether it's New Year's or just a night out, there *is* such a thing as too much sparkle (the fringe, the sheer).
- The boots-and-hat combo are too cowgirls-gone-wild.

IS IT A DO OR A DON'T?

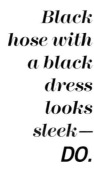

Black hose with a black dress looks sleek— DO.

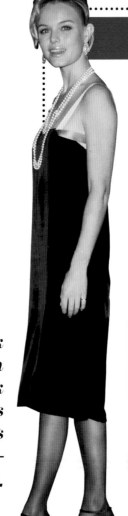

DON'T *overdo the flower trend.*

PANTYHOSE

These days stockings are back, and we're happy: Sometimes your legs get cold! Just stick to black or smoke-colored ones, which are always slimming, and wear with closed-toe shoes. (Opaque tights look fine with open toes, though.) Whatever you do, avoid candy-colored stockings—they're strictly for little girls.

OUR VERDICT: *a DO if done right*

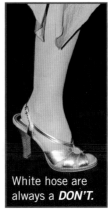

White hose are always a **DON'T.**

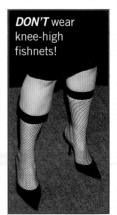

DON'T wear knee-high fishnets!

FLOWERS IN YOUR HAIR

A flower is a lovely hair accessory—just make sure to keep it simple. A single, delicate flower tucked behind your ear or into an updo looks elegant. Just DON'T overdo it with a flower that's too large and overpowering, or multiple flowers that turn your head into a centerpiece.

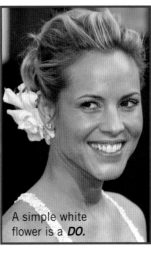

A simple white flower is a **DO.**

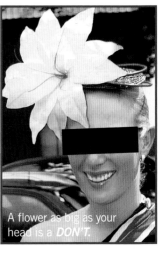

A flower as big as your head is a **DON'T.**

OUR VERDICT: *if they're huge, they're a DON'T*

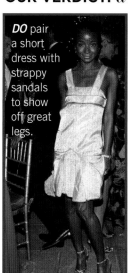

THE PASHMINA

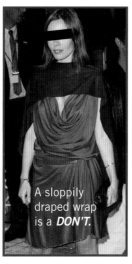

A sloppily draped wrap is a **DON'T.**

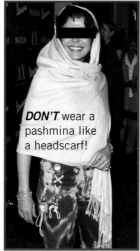

DON'T wear a pashmina like a headscarf!

Pashminas had their heyday in the late '90s, but they're worth hanging onto—they keep you warm on cool nights and work well with dressy attire. Black, brown and ivory are your best investments. Keep the look elegant by draping around your shoulders or low on your arms.

OUR VERDICT: *a DO if done right*

DO match your wrap to your dress for a streamlined look.

THE MINIDRESS

Wearing a short dress to a big event can be a DO as long as you keep the proportions right. Stick to styles that fall a few inches above the knee, and know that *looser* shapes, as at right, look more chic than skintight minis.

OUR VERDICT: *a DO—but keep it tasteful*

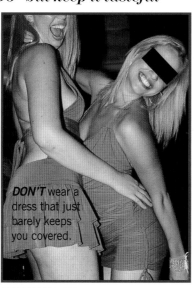

DO pair a short dress with strappy sandals to show off great legs.

DON'T wear a dress that just barely keeps you covered.

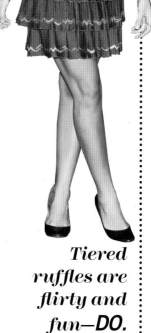

Tiered ruffles are flirty and fun—DO.

ALWAYS **A DON'T** FOR SPECIAL EVENTS

Big, overdone hair

Sequin overload

Anything sheer . . . with nothing underneath

Microminis

Flip-flops

Mesh

Ratty denim

Heels that are too high and/ or painful to dance in

Too much bling

"TAKE ME FROM FRUMPY TO SEXY!"

This concert harpist knows all about dressing for special events but admits she slipped up on the outfit below: "I bought this on a recent trip to Ireland because I thought the skirt was really pretty, but I had a hard time finding a top to go with it. I chose this camisole out of desperation, and now I think it makes me look frumpy and like I OD'd on satin and lace!" An easy fix: Just concentrate on one great piece that shows off your favorite body part. Done!

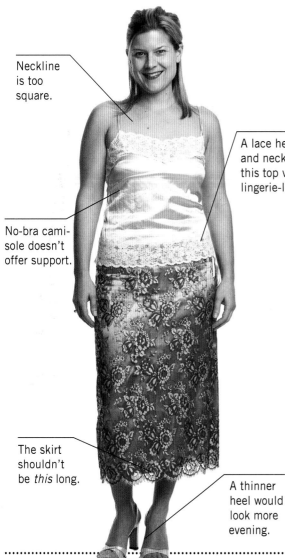

Delicate earrings dress up outfit.

Scoopneck shows a *hint* of cleavage.

Neckline is too square.

A lace hem and neck make this top very lingerie-like.

No-bra camisole doesn't offer support.

Empire-waist shirt puts focus on her narrow ribcage.

The skirt shouldn't be *this* long.

A thinner heel would look more evening.

Bright pattern steers eyes toward her upper body.

Sleek pants make for long-looking legs.

Strappy sandals—fun!

BEFORE:
Kirsten Agresta, 36

OUTDOOR CONCERT
"This fits me in all the places I like to emphasize and flatters even those I don't."

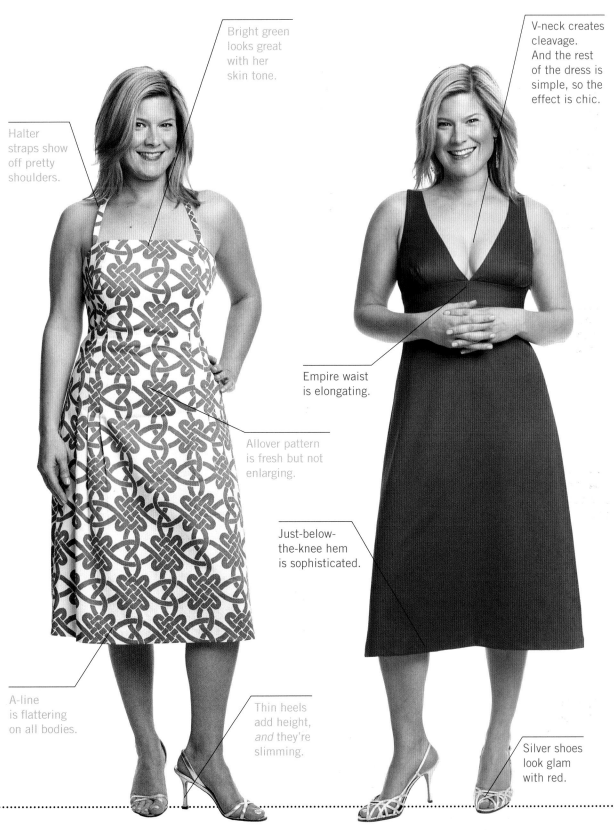

Bright green looks great with her skin tone.

Halter straps show off pretty shoulders.

Allover pattern is fresh but not enlarging.

A-line is flattering on all bodies.

Thin heels add height, *and* they're slimming.

V-neck creates cleavage. And the rest of the dress is simple, so the effect is chic.

Empire waist is elongating.

Just-below-the-knee hem is sophisticated.

Silver shoes look glam with red.

COCKTAILS AT A GALLERY

"A fun, flirty dress that makes me look not too serious."

LAUNCH PARTY

"It gives me cleavage I never knew I had— and it makes me feel sexy and hot!"

"MAKE ME LOOK ELEGANT!"

"My friend talked me into this dress," says Felicia about her "before" outfit. "She said I should show off my legs! Maybe it's a bit much?" It is—but only because the mini length makes the *rest* of her great body look out of proportion. This editorial assistant's style is "urban mixed with classic. I'm eclectic but not eccentric!" She doesn't need to try so hard to make jaws drop—it's much more polished to be lower-key.

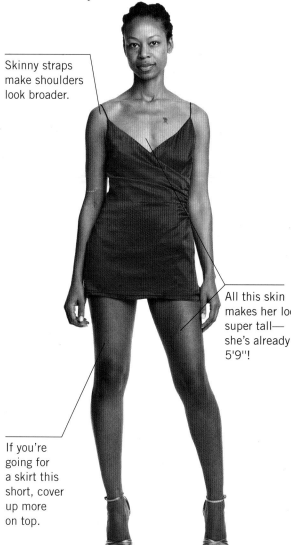

A boatneck is universally flattering.

Bejeweled neckline is pretty without being overwhelming.

Skinny straps make shoulders look broader.

Fitted shift skims her curves nicely.

All this skin makes her look super tall—she's already 5'9"!

If you're going for a skirt this short, cover up more on top.

Two-inch heels are all she needs.

BEFORE:
Felicia Dunston, 27

HOLIDAY PARTY
"The jewels around the collar give a dressier look without being old-ladyish."

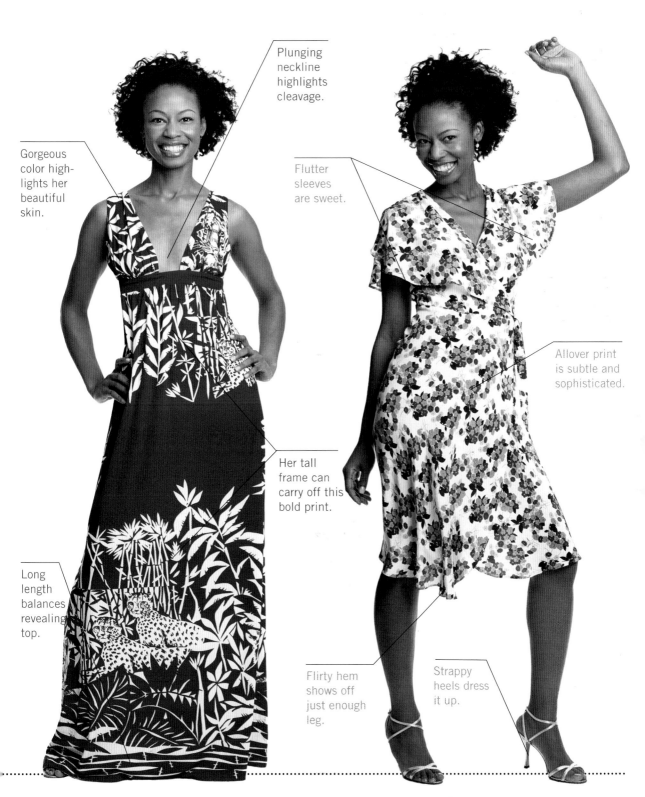

Plunging neckline highlights cleavage.

Gorgeous color highlights her beautiful skin.

Flutter sleeves are sweet.

Allover print is subtle and sophisticated.

Her tall frame can carry off this bold print.

Long length balances revealing top.

Flirty hem shows off just enough leg.

Strappy heels dress it up.

EVENING WEDDING

"I love the 1970s vintage look and low-cut neckline. I look like my mother in her prime!"

SUNDAY CHURCH

"This is a very ladylike dress, while still being comfortable and easy to wear."

"I WANT TO FLATTER MY CURVES!"

Rebecca's voluptuous figure doesn't deserve to be covered up in this shapeless dress. "I wore this for New Year's Eve," she says. "Sometimes it's easier to find something like this than a dress that fits really well." Not so! By highlighting Rebecca's best features—her waist, décolletage and amazing smile— she gets a great, non-mumsy look for any event. After this makeover she said, "Curves are good—I'll never cover them up again!"

A fuller face looks best with fuller hair—the proportion's right.

Halter top shows off a bit of cleavage.

Beading at neckline draws the eye in.

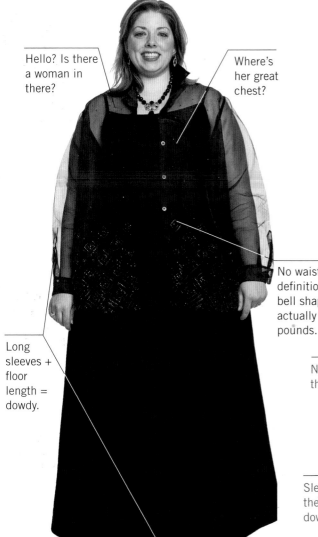

Hello? Is there a woman in there?

Where's her great chest?

No waist definition and bell shape actually *add* pounds.

Nicely fitted through waist.

Long sleeves + floor length = dowdy.

Sleek all the way down!

BEFORE:
Rebecca Mazzarella, 28

BLACK-TIE WEDDING

"I feel really glamorous in this dress. It's not the cover-me-up black dress you see on so many plus-size women."

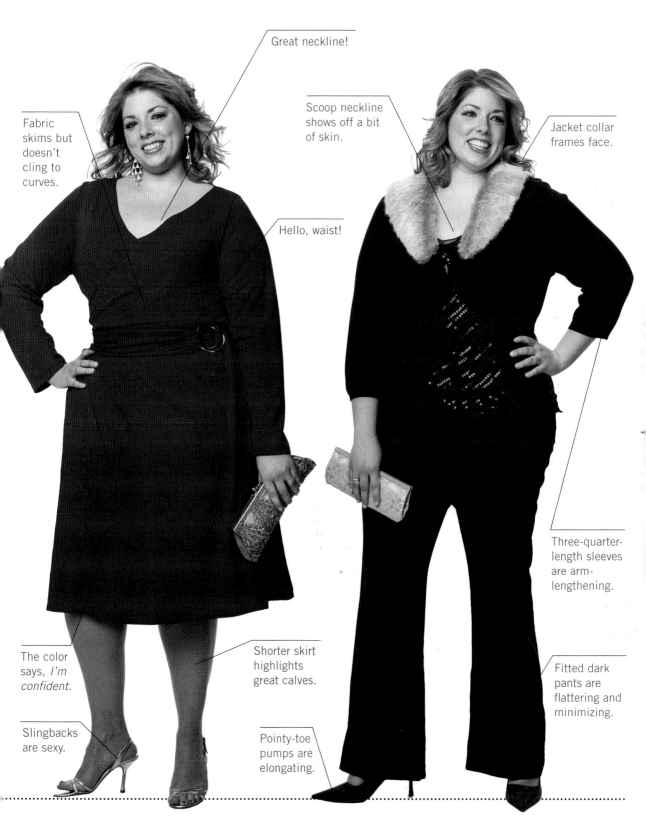

Great neckline!

Scoop neckline shows off a bit of skin.

Fabric skims but doesn't cling to curves.

Jacket collar frames face.

Hello, waist!

Three-quarter-length sleeves are arm-lengthening.

The color says, *I'm confident.*

Shorter skirt highlights great calves.

Fitted dark pants are flattering and minimizing.

Slingbacks are sexy.

Pointy-toe pumps are elongating.

ART SHOW

"This is my LRD—'Little Red Dress'! It highlights my smaller waist, and the deep V-neck keeps the focus on my face."

ANNIVERSARY DINNER

"I'm not used to wearing such form-fitting clothes, but this really flatters me. It feels very Audrey Hepburn."

THE 20 *WORST* DON'TS OF ALL TIME!

Here, in descending order, are the fashion faux pas our roving photographer sees most often. Committed one of these sins? Committed ten? Relax— you're not alone.

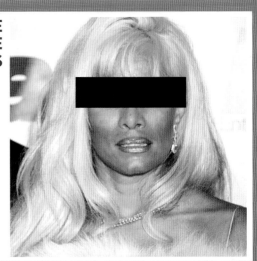

19
WORK CLOTHES WITH SNEAKERS

TOO MUCH BLING

20

18

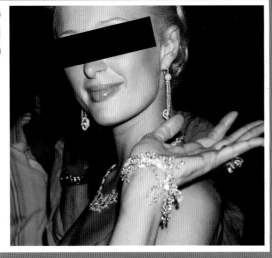

BUTT CLEAVAGE

ORANGE FAKE TANS

17

RUDE MESSAGE T-SHIRTS

16

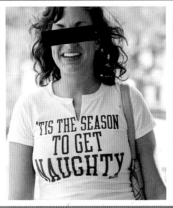

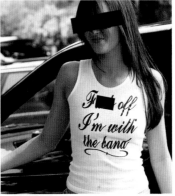

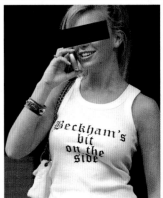

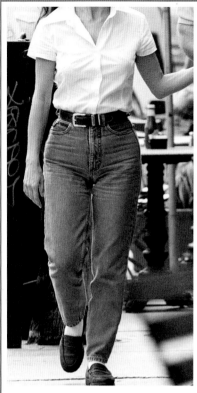

"MOM" JEANS

15

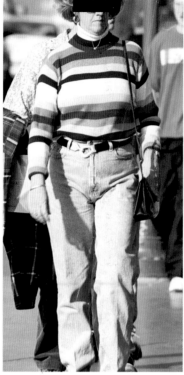

TOO-SHORT SKIRTS AND SHORTS

14

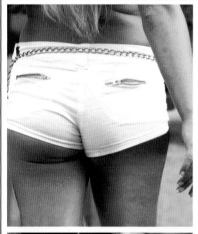

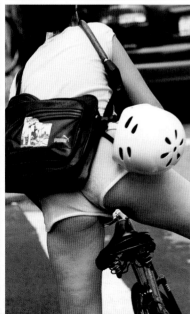

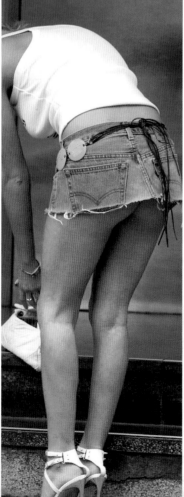

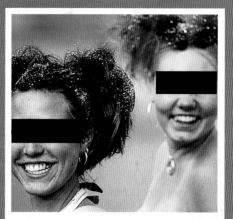

CANDY-COLORED HAIR

13

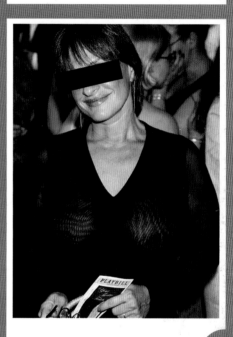

SEE-THROUGH CLOTHES

12

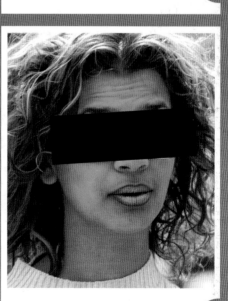

VISIBLE LIP LINER

11

continues...

THE
20 *WORST*
DON'TS
OF ALL TIME!

...continued **8**

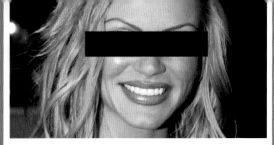

**OVERLY
TWEEZED
EYEBROWS**

10

SCRUNCHIES, BANANA CLIPS AND OTHER EXTREME HAIR ACCESSORIES

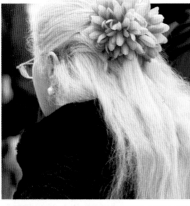

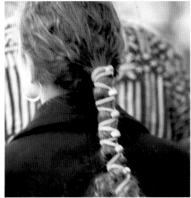

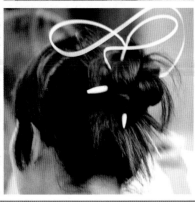

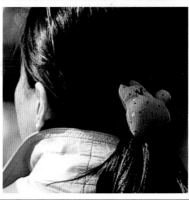

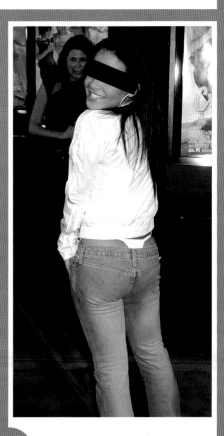

7

**THONGS
ON DISPLAY**

**WEIRD
HEADGEAR**

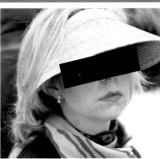

**TOO-
TIGHT
CLOTHES
(OUCH!)**

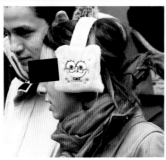

9

6

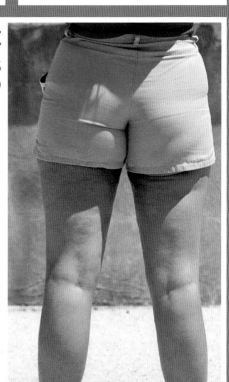

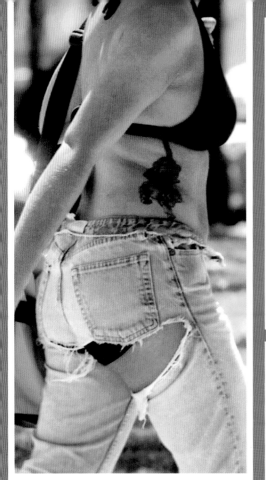

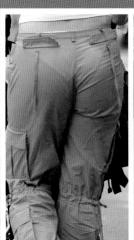
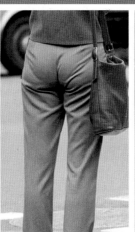

THE
NO-BRA LOOK

3

ANYTHING
MESH

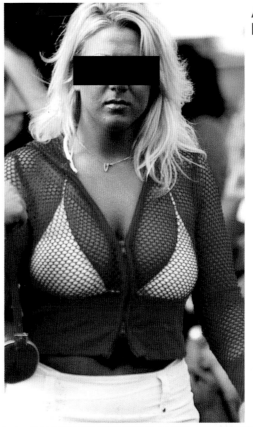

HOLEY
DENIM

5

BIG
HAIR

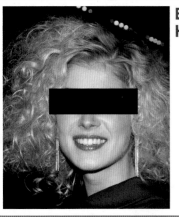

4

2

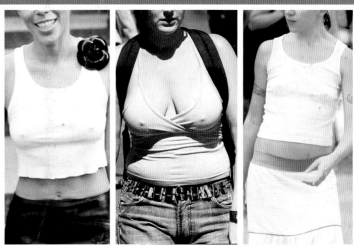
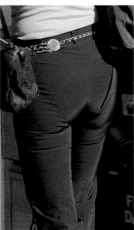
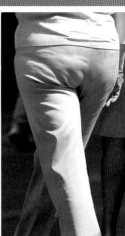

VISIBLE
PANTY
LINES

1

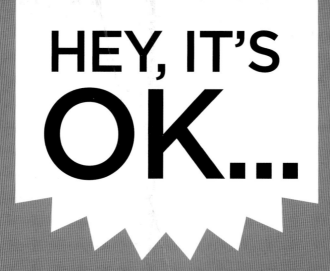

HEY, IT'S OK...

Every woman has those days when she stands in front of her closet, says, "The hell with it!" and puts on exactly what she feels like wearing. And those are often the days you look best. Long live rule-breaking! We say it's perfectly fine...

TO **IGNORE** ANY AND ALL "IT" **TRENDS.**

• • •

TO **HAVE A PONYTAIL** BE YOUR "LOOK."

• • •

TO **FEEL** MASSIVELY **ANNOYED** THAT NO TWO BRANDS' SIZE 2s OR 12s OR 20s EVER FIT THE SAME.

• • •

TO HEAR YOUR MOM'S VOICE SAYING **"YOU'RE WEARING THAT?"** AND WEAR IT ANYWAY.

• • •

TO **PAIR A** FANCY DESIGNER **SKIRT WITH A** WHITE **MEN'S TANK** TOP FROM THE DRUGSTORE.

• • •

TO **FEEL CONFLICTED** ABOUT FUR.

TO **WALK OUT ON
ANY SALESPERSON** WHO
DOESN'T SEEM TO WANT YOUR BUSINESS.

• • •

TO **OVERDRESS FOR
WORK**, JUST TO KEEP THEM GUESSING.

• • •

TO **KEEP YOUR
EX-BOYFRIEND'S**
UNMATCHABLY COZY **XXL SWEATER**
(AND NOT TELL HIS SUCCESSOR HOW YOU
CAME TO OWN SUCH A THING).

• • •

TO **SHOW UP DRESSED
TO THE HILT** KNOWING EVERYONE
ELSE WILL BE IN JEANS—IN FACT, *BECAUSE*
THEY'LL ALL BE IN JEANS.

• • •

TO **GET MARRIED IN A**
SEXY **RED DRESS.**

• • •

TO NOT **WASH YOUR
HAIR** EVERY DAY. OR EVEN **EVERY
OTHER DAY.**

• • •

TO **PAY BIG MONEY
FOR THINGS YOU LOVE** AND
SMALL MONEY FOR EVERYTHING ELSE.

glossary

ANKLE BITERS \'an-kəl 'bī-ters\ *a Don't:* Also known as *floods* or *waders.* Pants that are too short, visually chopping off the length of your leg. Unflattering; avoid 'em.

·······································

BACK BOOB \'bak 'büb\ *a Don't:* That unsightly back-flesh bulging you get from ill-fitting bras and/or too-tight tops or strapless dresses. Easily remedied if you buy what fits.

·······································

BEDHEAD \'bed 'hed\ *can be a Do or a Don't:* Done unintentionally, describes unbrushed, matted, askew hair. Done intentionally, describes time-consuming, product-enhanced style that is sexily tousled and, yes, a Do.

·······································

BLING \'bling\ *can be a Do or a Don't:* Any jumbo-scale, massive-wattage jewelry, worn by man or woman, that's impossible not to notice. Used appropriately, can dress up an outfit and look luxe; used inappropriately and in mass amounts, can make you look like the Vegas Strip.

·······································

BUTT CLEAVAGE \'bət 'klē-vij\ *a Don't:* Also *coin slot* and *plumber butt.* The ubiquitous visible-crack syndrome created by low-rise jeans and equally low-rise underwear, or an absence thereof. Particularly common when bending over.

·······································

CHOO SHOES \'chü 'shüz\ *a Do:* Any expensive, killer high heels that make you feel like hot sex on a platter every time you wear them. From Jimmy Choo, maker of this kind of gorgeous footwear.

·······································

COCKTAIL ATTIRE \'käk-tāl ə-'tī(-ə)r\ Commonly seen on invitations. Means dressy, but not black-tie dressy. Confused? Wear your *LBD* (see below).

·······································

CREATIVE BLACK TIE \krē-'ā-tiv 'blak 'tī\ More invitation lingo. Means formal attire with a nontraditional twist, i.e., a ball-gown skirt with white menswear shirt.

·······································

CUTLETS \'kət-lətz\ *can be a Do or a Don't:* Thin, rubbery bust enhancers resembling raw chicken cutlets. Slipped into a bra, they add volume and lift, in much the same way as a push-up bra. Secure with double-stick tape to prevent *Wardrobe Malfunction* (see below).

DUMPSTER CHIC \'dəm(p)-stər 'shēk\ *a Don't:* A hobo/waif-like, Salvation Army–style look, displayed by the Olsen twins on the streets of New York City during their freshman year of college. Components often include aged cowboy boots; supersized sweaters; ripped tights; long peasant skirts; baggy tunics; and giant sunglasses—frequently worn all at the same time, and while carrying a $3,000 purse.

·······································

ELEPHANT ANKLES \'e-lə-fənt 'an-kəls\ *a Don't:* A condition caused by sagging stockings, tights or socks that wrinkle at the ankles.

·······································

FESTIVE ATTIRE \'fes-tiv ə-'tī(-ə)r\ More confusing invitation-speak. Denotes semi-formal clothing with a party flair. When in doubt, wear a piece with sparkle.

·······································

GWYNETH JEANS \'gwin-eth jēnz\ *a Do:* Jeans that fit you perfectly, as if quite literally made for you; named for Blue Cult's Gwyneth jeans, designed with Ms. Paltrow in mind.

·······································

THE "IT" {INSERT ITEM} \thē 'it\ *a Do... for the moment:* Usually an accessory, such as a bag or shoe, that has been deemed by mysterious and invisible fashion forces to be the must-have item of the season. Alas, virtually guaranteed to be over and replaced by some other "It" within six months.

·······································

LBD \'el 'bē 'dē\ *a Do:* An abbreviation for the Little Black Dress, an eternal Do that can cover you wherever you're going. Flattering and (especially in a not-too-casual fabric) hugely versatile.

·······································

MOM JEANS \'mäm jēnz\ *a Don't:* No offense, Mom. Jeans characterized by one or all of the following: tapered ankles, high waist, pleats. (As parodied on *Saturday Night Live:* "Because you're not a woman anymore—you're a mom!") Better choices for *all* women: lower (but not *too* low) waists, boot cuts.

·······································

MONO BOOB \'mä-nō 'büb\ *a Don't (but hard to avoid):* Also *uniboob.* Two breasts that look like one, caused by the smooshing, shelflike effect of a sports bra. A necessary evil for achieving support while working out.

SOME **DOS & DON'TS** ARE SO COMMON THEY EARN THEIR OWN PLACE IN OUR FASHION VOCABULARY. HERE'S STYLE SLANG EVERY WELL-INFORMED WOMAN SHOULD KNOW:

MUFFIN TOP \'mə-fən 'täp\ *a Don't:*
The hip and stomach bulge created when too-tight, too-low jeans force your flesh to bubble over the top of the waistband. Can occur on every body type, even the fittest. Concealable with the help of a long top.

PHONY PONY \'fō-nē 'pō-nē\ *can be a Do or a Don't:* Attachable hair extension designed to turn a puny pony into a thick and believable tail. Ingenious, but wear with caution: They can, and do, fall out.

THE RACHEL ZOE EFFECT \thē 'ra-chül 'zō-ā i-'fekt\ *a Don't:* The look popularized by celeb stylist Zoe, who dresses Lindsay Lohan, Nicole Richie and others in huge sunglasses, jeans tucked into boots, layered tees, multiple necklaces, and an "It" bag (see above). But watch out: Follow *any* celeb look too closely, and you'll be a Don't.

RIGHT-HAND RING \'rīt-hand 'ring\ *a Do:*
The new trend (started by celebs and endorsed by big jewelry companies) of women buying their *own* diamond rings—and wearing them on their right hands, to denote independence.

THE SATC EFFECT AND SJP \'es ā tē sē\ *can be a Do or a Don't:* Short for the popular HBO show *Sex and the City*, and its star, Sarah Jessica Parker. The fashion shown on the series influenced women around the country to wear assertively girly items and uber-trendy outfits such as name-plate necklaces, high heels with shorts, black bras with white shirts, tutus and other attire generally considered "fabulous" by its younger audience and "ridiculous" by an older demographic.

SCRUNCHIE \'skrən-chē\ *a Don't:* A bulky, fabric-covered elastic hair band, popular in the big-hair era of the late eighties and early nineties. Save it for washing your face.

SKUNK HAIR \'skənk 'her\ *a Don't:* Hair color characterized by highly contrasting stripes or highlights, resulting in a skunklike appearance.

SPANX® \'spankz\ *a Do:* A brand of new-generation body-shaping undergarments (thankfully bearing no resemblance to your grandmother's girdle), enabling normal-size women to look paparazzi-ready in bare and form-fitting clothes.

TANOREXIC \'ta-nə-'rek-sik\ *a Don't:* A person set on maintaining a deep, dark, year-round tan by any means necessary: tanning beds, self-tanning creams, spray-on tanning booths, and of course, sun exposure. Tanorexia lifetime achievement award goes to actor George Hamilton.

TOE CLEAVAGE \'tō 'klē-vij\ *a Do:*
Exposed spot on the top of the foot where the toes begin, created by (generally quite sexy) shoes with a low vamp.

UGGS \'əgz\ *can be a Do or a Don't:* Brand of sheepskin boots that reached cult status after all of Hollywood began wearing them in the early 21st century, most commonly at Sundance. Still irresistibly comfortable but, like all "It" items, outdated. Wear yours on covert cappuccino runs—or when it's really snowy.

UNDERBOOBS \'ən-dər 'bübz\ *a Don't:*
Exposure of the underfold of the breast. Most often the result of too-small bikini tops.

VPL \'vē 'pē 'el\ *a Don't:* Abbreviation for Visible Panty Line; and the reason thongs had to be invented. Clingy, tight fabrics dramatically increase incidence of this problem. Prevent with a quick, 360-degree mirror check before leaving home.

WARDROBE MALFUNCTION \'wór-drōb mal-'fən(k)-shən\ *a Don't, but not your fault:* The delicious term coined by Justin Timberlake after Janet Jackson's shirt "mistakenly" exposed her breast at the Super Bowl. Use this phrase to defend yourself in the wake of your *own* Don't moments.

WEDGIE \'we-jē\ *a Don't:* A condition wherein pants get stuck in a wickedly uncomfortable position. Most commonly seen in too-small pants or in very loose ones made of flimsy material.

PHOTO CREDITS

ON-THE-STREET PHOTOGRAPHY BY RONNIE ANDREN
MAKEOVER PHOTOGRAPHY BY MARC ROYCE

Inside front cover: Ronnie Andren [RA]; p. 2: RA; p.4: RA; p. 6: Courtesy Cindi Leive; p. 7: Nathan Sayers; p. 8: Courtesy Cindi Leive (2); timeline image: Nathan Sayers; p. 9: Nathan Sayers (2); p. 10: Donato Sardella/WireImage.com; timeline images: Nathan Sayers (3); p. 11 (top): RA; (bottom): Chance Yeh/Patrick McMullan;

BODY BASICS pp. 16–17: RA (2); p. 21: Anthony Dixon/LFI; p. 23: Roger Karnbad/CelebrityPhoto.com; p. 25: Axelle/Bauer-Griffin.com; p. 27: Dimitrios Kambouris/WireImage.com; p. 29: Paul Smith/Featureflash/Retna; p. 32 (clockwise from top left): Janet Gough/CelebrityPhoto.com, RA(2), Jason Kirk/Eric Ford/Online USA/Getty Images, RA (3); p. 33 (clockwise from top left): RA (3), JS Turgeon/INFGoff.com, RA;

YOUR WEEKEND LIFE p. 34: Mark Leibowitz; p. 35: RA; pp. 38-39 (left–right): RA, Mark Allan/Alpha/Globe Photos, Fame Pictures, RA (2); p. 40 (clockwise from top): RA, Dimitrios Kambouris/WireImage.com, The Kobal Collection, RA(5); p. 41 (clockwise from top): RA (7), Ray Mickshaw/WireImage.com, RA (2); p. 43 (top row, left to right): RA, Katie Lee Arrowsmith/Splash News, RA; (center row, left to right): Nancy Kaszerman/Zuma Press, RA(2); (bottom row, left to right): Mark Leibowitz, RA, Steve Granitz/WireImage.com; (right column, from top): RA (4); p. 45 (top row, left to right): RA, Bauer-Griffin.com, Riquet/Bauer-Griffin.com; (center row, left to right): George Pimentel/WireImage.com, RA (2); (bottom row, left to right): RA, Mark Leibowitz, RA; (right column, from top): RA (4); p. 47 (top row, left to right): RA, Mark Leibowitz, Matrix/Bauer-Griffin.com; (center row, left to right): Rachid/Chris/Bauer-Griffin.com, Jean-Paul Aussenard/WireImage.com, Lawrence Lucier/FilmMagic.com; (bottom row, left to right): Mark Leibowitz, Chris Weeks/WireImage.com, RA; (right column, from top): London Entertainment/Splash News, Blanco/X17-agency.com, RA (2); p. 49: (top row, left to right): RA, Green/Heining/INFGoff.com, RA; (center row, left to right): Lawrence Schwartzwald/Splash News, RA (2); (bottom row, left to right): RA, Frank Olsen/startraksphoto.com, RA; (right column, from top): RA (2), Mark Sullivan/WireImage.com, RA; p. 51: (top row, left to right): Limelight Pictures, RA(2); (center row, left to right): RA (2), JFX/X17agency.com; (bottom row, left to right): Gregory Pace/FilmMagic.com, RA (2); (right column, from top): RA (4); pp. 52–53 (left–right): RA (5); p. 54 (clockwise from top left): RA (6); p. 55 (clockwise from top left): Getty Images, Flynet Pictures, The Kobal Collection, RA, Richard Beetham/Chris Pittam/Splash News; (right column, from top): RA (4); p. 56 (from top): Dave Benett/Getty Images, Carlos Alvarez/Getty Images, RA; p. 57: (top row, left to right): Frederick M. Brown/Getty Images, RA, Jonathan Friolo/IHP/Splash News; (center row, left to right): Fpix/Bauer-Griffin.com, RA (2); (bottom row, left to right): RA (3); (right column, from top): RA (4); pp. 58–59 (top row, left to right): RA (3); (bottom row, left to right): Gregg DeGuire/WireImage.com, Dave M. Benett/Getty Images, RA (3); pp. 60–61: RA (all); pp. 62–63 (left to right): RA (2), Rex Features, RA; p. 64–65 (left to right): RA (2), Mark Leibowitz, RA; 66 (clockwise from top left): Matt Baron/BEImages, RA (2), Mike Webster/Rex Features, London Entertainment/Splash; p. 67 (clockwise from top left): RA (3), Zasi/Bauer-Griffin.com, RA (2); pp. 74-75: RA (all);

YOUR WORK LIFE pp. 76–77: RA (2); pp. 80–81 (left to right): RA, Luis Guerra/Ramey Photo, RA (3); p. 82 (clockwise from top left): Arnaldo Magnani/Getty Images, Vince Bucci/Getty Images, Donato Sardella/WireImage.com, Lalo Yasky/WireImage.com, RA (2); p. 83 (left column, from top): Guerci Gros/X17agency.com, Michael Loccisano/FilmMagic.com, RA, Jennifer Graylock/JPIstudios.com; (second column, from top: RA (4); (Third column, from top): Dan Callister/Pacificcoastnews.com, RA; (Right column, from top): RA (4); p. 84–85 (left to right): RA (3), Sylvain Gaboury/DMIPhoto.com, RA; p. 87 (top row, left to right): RA (3); (center row, left to right): RA, ViPix/Abacusa.com, RA; (bottom row, left to right): Stewart Cook/Rex Features, RA (2); (right column, from top): RA (4); page 88 (clockwise from top left): Michael Caulfield/Wire-Image.com, Everett Collection, Donato Sardella/WireImage.com, RA (4); p. 89 (clockwise from top left): RA, Gregg DeGuire/WireImage.com, RA (3); (right column, from top: RA (4); p. 91 (top row, left to right): Jean-Paul Aussenard/Wireimage.com, RA (2); (center row, left to right): Tony Barson/Wireimage.com, RA (2); (bottom row, left to right): RA (3); (right column, from top): RA (4); p. 93 (top row, left to right): RA (3); (center row, left to right): RA, George Pimentel/WireImage.com, RA; (bottom row, left to right): RA (3); (right column, from top): RA (4); pp. 94–95 (left to right): RA, Patsy Lynch/Retna Ltd., RA (3); Page 96 (clockwise from top left): Barry King/Wireimage.com, Sonia Moskowitz/Globe Photos, Steve Eichner/Women's Wear Daily, Jim Smeal/WireImage.com, RA (2), Anthony Harvey/Getty Images, Ron Galella/WireImage.com; p. 97 (clockwise from top left): Jim Spellman/WireImage.com, Andreas Rentz/Getty Images, MPTV.net, RA, Flynetpictures.com, RA; (right column, from top): RA (4); p. 99 (top row, left to right): RA (3); (center row, left to right): RA, Ginsburg-Spaly/X17agency.com, RA; (bottom row, left to right): RA (3); (right column, from top): RA (4); p. 100 (top to bottom): RA (2), Katie Lee Arrowsmith/Splash News; p. 101: RA (all); p. 102 (top to bottom): RA (2), Punchstock; p. 103: RA (all); p. 104: RA (all); p. 105: RA (all); p. 106–107 (left to right): RA (2), Richard Young/Rex Features, RA; p. 108–109 (left to right): RA (2), Anthony Dixon/LFI, RA; p. 110 (clockwise from top left): Mark Leibowitz, Henry McGee/Globe Photos, RA (3) p. 111 (clockwise from top left): RA (3), Frazer Harrison/Getty Images, RA; p. 118 (clockwise from top left): RA (5); p. 119 (clockwise from top left): Lisa Rose/JPI, RA, David Westing/Getty Images, RA;

YOUR NIGHTS OUT p. 120–121 RA (2); p. 124–125 (left to right): RA, Sean Gallup/Getty Images, Axelle/Bauer-Griffin.com, RA, Mark Mainz/Getty Images; p. 126 (clockwise from top left): Mike Marsland/WireImage.com, Lester Cohen/WireImage.com, Ruy Sanchez Blanco, Mark Leibowitz, Jesse Grant/WireImage.com, Paul Smith/Featureflash/Retna; p. 127 (left column, from top): Axelle/Bauer-Griffin.com, Charles Sykes/Rex Features, Mike Guastella/WireImage.com, Gregg DeGuire/WireImage.com; (second column, from top): RA, Jen Lowery/LFI, Tim Whitby/WireImage.com, RA; (third column, from top): Mark Leibowitz, George Pimentel/WireImage.com, RA (far right column, from top): Peter Kramer/Getty Images, RA (2), Stewart Cook/Rex; pp. 128–129 (left to right): Stewart Cook/Rex, John Shearer/WireImage.com, Gregg DeGuire/WireImage.com, Jen Lowery/LFI, Jonathan Friolo/IHP/Splash News; (clockwise from top left): Stephen Lovekin/FilmMagic.com, Robin Platzer/FilmMagic.com, Michael Buckner/Getty Images, Jean-Paul Aussenard/WireImage.com, RA (5); p. 131 (clockwise from top left): Nicolas Khayat/Abacausa.com, Steve Kondilis/Bauer-Griffin.com, Amanda Edwards/Getty Images, Peter Kramer/Getty Images (2), Stuart Atkins/Rex Features, Rex Features, Jill Johnson/JPI, Ron Galella/WireImage.com; (right column, from top): Tsuni/Gamma, Larry Busacca/WireImage.com, Tony Barson/WireImage.com, Ron Galella/WireImage.com; pp. 132–133: (left to right): Michael Buckner/Getty Images, Lawrence Lucier/FilmMagic.com, RA (2), Dimitrios Kambouris/WireImage.com; p. 134 (clockwise from top left): Brenda Chase, Kevin Mazur/Wire-Image.com, Roger Karnbad/CelebrityPhoto.com, Frederick M. Brown/Getty Image, Mark Leibowitz, RA, Dave Lewis/Rex USA; p.135 (clockwise from top left): Carlos Alvarez/Getty Images, John Ricard/FilmMagic.com, Dimitrios Kambouris/WireImage.com, Globe Photos, RA, Mark Leibowitz; (right column, from top): Dave Benett/Getty Images, Gregg DeGuire/WireImage.com, RA (2); p. 136 (clockwise from left): Jean-Paul Aussenard/WireImage.com, Djamilla Rosa Cochran/WireImage.com, Jeff Kravitz/FilmMagic.com, Arun Nevader/FilmMagic.com, RA, Tsuni/Gamma; p. 137 (clockwise from top left): James Devaney/WireImage.com, Kevin Mazur/WireImage.com, Jeff Vespa/WireImage.com, Dimitrios Kambouris/WireImage.com, RA, Theo Wargo/WireImage.com, Kevin Mazur/WireImage.com, RA(2); p. 138 (from top): RA (all); p. 139 (top row, left to right): Axelle/Bauer-Griffin.com, RA (2); (center row, left to right): RA (2), Erik C Pendzich/Rex Features; (bottom row, left to right): RA, Brian Prahl/Splash News, RA; (right column, from top): Gene Blevins/Corbis, RA (3); p. 140 (from top: Lisa O'Connor/Zuma Press, Anna Pocaro/LEP/Splash News, Dave Benett/Getty Images; p. 141 (top row, left to right): Tsuni/Gamma, RA (2); (center row, left to right): Marsaili McGrath/Getty Images, Frazer Harrison/Getty Images, RA; (bottom row, left to right): Jeff Vespa/WireImage.com, RA, Lisa O'Connor/Zuma Press; (right column, from top): RA, Vincent Kessler/Reuters/Corbis, Mike Valdez/Zuma/Corbis, John Schults/Reuters/Corbis; pp. 142¬–143 (left to right): Lester Cohen/WireImage.

com, Mark Leibowitz, RA, Can Nguyen/LFI; pp. 144–145 (left to right): Gregory Pace/FilmMagic.com, RA (2), Michael Williams/LFI; p. 146 (clockwise from left): Michael Loccisano/FilmMagic.com, Theo Wargo/WireImage.com, Jason Kirk/Newsmakers/Getty Images, RA; p. 147: (top row, left to right): Araldo Di Crollalanza/Rex Features, Tony Barson/WireImage.com, Djamilla Rosa Cochran/WireImage.com; (center row, left to right): Djamilla Rosa Cochran/WireImage.com, Pascal Le Segretain/Getty Images, Mike Guastella/WireImage.com; (bottom row, left to right): RA (2), Dimitrios Kambouris/WireImage.com; pp. 154–155: RA (all);

YOUR SPECIAL EVENTS p. 156: Jon Kopaloff/FilmMagic.com; p. 157: Amanda Edwards/Getty Images for Chopard; p.161 (top row, left to right): Alberto Tamargo/Getty Images, David Fisher/LFI, Alec Michael/Globe Photos; (center row, left to right): Evan Agostini/Getty Images, Michael Williams/LFI, George Pimentel/WireImage.com; (bottom row, left to right): Henry McGee/Globe Photos, Steve Granitz/Wireimage.com, Gregg De-Guire/WireImage.com; (right column, from top): Pascal Le Segretain/Getty Images, Jason Winslow/Splash News; p. 163 (top row, left to right): Robin Platzer/FilmMagic.com, Jon Kopaloff/FilmMagic.com, James Smeal/Ron Galella; (center row, left to right): Tim Whitby/WireImage.com, Gilbert Flores/CelebrityPhoto.com, Henry McGee/Globe Photos; (bottom row, left to right): Axelle/Bauer-Griffin.com, Tsuni/Gamma, Peter Kramer/Getty Images; (right column, from top): Showbiz Ireland/Getty Images, Steve Granitz/WireImage.com, Jean-Paul Aussenard/WireImage.com, Stewart Cook/Rex Features; p. 165 (top row, left to right): Jim Smeal/BEImages, Theo Wargo/WireImage.com, Paul McConnell/Getty Images; (center row, left to right): Jemal Countess/WireImage.com, Rebecca Sapp/WireImage.com, Tim Whitby/WireImage.com; (bottom row, left to right): Frank Trapper/Corbis, Dimitrios Kambouris/WireImage.com, Gregg DeGuire/WireImage.com; (right column, from top): Trapper Frank/Corbis Sygma, Mark Mainz/Getty Images, Kevin Mazur/WireImage.com; p. 166 (from top): Arnaldo Magnani/Getty Images, RA, Pascal Le Segretain/Getty Images; p. 167 (top row, left to right): Bauer-Griffin, Jean Baptiste Lacroix/WireImage.com, Lisa Rose/JPIstudios.com; (center row, left to right): RA, Mark Mainz/Getty Images, RA; (bottom row, left to right): Gregory Pace/FilmMagic.com, Lisa O'Connor/Zuma/Corbis, Stephen Shugerman/Getty Images; (right column, from top): Daniele Venturelli/WireImage.com, Roger Karnbad/Celebrity-Photo.com, Steve Finn/Getty Images, Stephen Shugerman/Getty Images; p. 168 (from top): Sean Gallup/Getty Images, Thomas Lau/CelebrityPhoto.com, Dimitrios Kambouris/WireImage.com; p. 169 (top row, left to right): Berliner Studio/BEImages, Evan Agostini/Getty Images, Gilbert Flores/CelebrityPhoto.com; (center row, left to right): Jill Johnson/JPIstudios.com, David Livingston/Getty Images, Toby Melville/Reuters/Corbis; (bottom row, left to right): Lester Cohen/WireImage.com, Andrew H. Walker/Getty Images, Jill Johnson/JPIstudios.com; (right column, from top): Jim Smeal/BEImages, Lawrence Lucier/FilmMagic.com, James Quinton/WireImage.com, Jill Johnson/jpistudios.com; pp. 170–171 (left to right): Gregory Pace/FilmMagic.com, Steve Granitz/Wireimage.com, Kevin Winter/Getty Images, MJ Kim/Getty Images; pp. 172–173 (left to right): Sam Levi/WireImage.com, Jon Kopaloff/FilmMagic.com, Matrix/Bauer-Griffin.com, Rodrigo Varela/WireImage.com; p. 174 (clockwise from left): Mirek Towski/DMI/Time Life Pictures/Getty Images, Dimitrios Kambouris/WireImage.com, RA, Jo Hale/Getty Images, Capital Pictures, Jeff Vespa/WireImage.com; p. 175 (clockwise from top left): Chris Weeks/WireImage.com, Tony Barson/WireImage.com, Steve Granitz/WireImage.com, Daniele Venturelli/WireImage.com, RA, Joe Schildhorn/Patrick McMullan.

p. 182 (clockwise from top left): INFGoff.com, RA, Jennifer Graylock/jpistudios.com, DS001/ZBP/Zuma Press, KG001/ZBP/Zuma Press, RA (2); p. 183 (clockwise from top left): RA (3), Henry McGee/Globe Photos, RA, DS001/694/ZBP/Zuma Press, RA (2); p. 184 (clockwise from top right): Albert L. Ortega/WireImage.com, Gregg DeGuire/WireImage.com, RA (7); p. 185 (clockwise from top left): RA (9), Jim Spellman/WireImage.com

SPECIAL THANKS:
CONDÉ NAST PUBLICATIONS
MARK REITER
DARYL CHEN
SUSAN GOODALL
EDITORS: Maryellen Gordon, Kim Bonnell, Ashley Baker, Lauren Smith Brody, Ellen Seidman
MAKEOVERS: Suze Yalof Schwartz, Marina Albright
FASHION: Sarah Meikle
DESIGN: Peter Hemmel
PHOTOGRAPHY: Ronnie Andren, Julie Stone, Lindsay Chandler-Alexander

AND THANKS TO:
Margarita Bertsos, Lauren Bradshaw, Jasher Brea, Stacy Cousino, Geoffrey Collins, Kelly Crook, Suzanne Donaldson, Sally Dorst, Felicia Dunston, Siobhan Fitzpatrick, Alison Ward Frank, Molly Janik Gulati, Jill Herzig, Ashley Horne, Sasha Iglehart, Xanthipi Joannides, Lynda Laux-Bachand, Sara Nelson, Michelle Pacht, Samantha Rosenthal, Leslie Russo, Holland Utley, Katty Van Itallie, Kate Ward, Jennifer Weinberg, Jensen Wheeler Wolfe and Christy Whitney

THIS BOOK WAS PRODUCED BY:

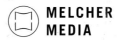

MELCHER
MEDIA

124 West 13th Street
New York, NY 10011
www.melcher.com

PUBLISHER: Charles Melcher
ASSOCIATE PUBLISHER: Bonnie Eldon
EDITOR IN CHIEF: Duncan Bock
PROJECT EDITOR: Megan Worman
ASSISTANT EDITOR: Lauren Nathan
PRODUCTION DIRECTOR: Andrea Hirsh

PHOTO EDITORS: Amelia Hennighausen, Julie Mihaly

DESIGNED BY: Number Seventeen, NYC

MELCHER MEDIA WISHES TO THANK:
Kyle Acebo, Jonathan Ambar, David E. Brown, Max J. Dickstein, Neil Egan, Jim Gaylord, Brian Herzig, E. Y. Lee, Lisa Maione, Joseph Manghise, Elise J. Marton, Janie Matthews, Mark J. Miller, Wendie Pecharsky, Lia Ronnen, Holly Rothman, Jessi Rymill, John Sanchez, Lindsey Stanberry, Alexandra Tart, Shoshana Thaler, Carl Williamson and Betty Wong

GOTHAM BOOKS, Published by Penguin Group (USA) Inc.,
375 Hudson Street, New York, New York 10014, U.S.A.

Penguin Group (Canada), 90 Eglinton Avenue East, Suite 700, Toronto,
Ontario M4P 2Y3, Canada (a division of Pearson Penguin Canada Inc.);
Penguin Books Ltd, 80 Strand, London WC2R 0RL, England; Penguin
Ireland, 25 St Stephen's Green, Dublin 2, Ireland (a division of Penguin
Books Ltd); Penguin Group (Australia), 250 Camberwell Road, Camber-
well, Victoria 3124, Australia (a division of Pearson Australia Group Pty
Ltd); Penguin Books India Pvt Ltd, 11 Community Centre, Panchsheel
Park, New Delhi - 110 017, India; Penguin Group (NZ), cnr Airborne
and Rosedale Roads, Albany, Auckland 1310, New Zealand (a division of
Pearson New Zealand Ltd); Penguin Books (South Africa) (Pty) Ltd, 24
Sturdee Avenue, Rosebank, Johannesburg 2196, South Africa

Penguin Books Ltd, Registered Offices:
80 Strand, London WC2R 0RL, England

Published by Gotham Books, a division of Penguin Group (USA) Inc.

First printing, September 2006
10 9 8 7 6 5 4 3 2 1

Gotham Books and the skyscraper logo are trademarks of Penguin Group
(USA) Inc.

Glamour and Dos & Don'ts are trademarks of Condé Nast Publications.

ISBN 1-592-40233-X

Printed in China